Management
of Labour
The Dublin Experience

21 Day

University of Plymouth Library
Subject to status this item may be renewed
via your Voyager account
http://voyager.plymouth.ac.uk
Tel: (01752) 232323

Univ

Subjec

http:/

Exe
Exmc
Plymou

D0230551

Commissioning Editor: *Stephanie Donley*
Project Development Manager: *Tim Kimber*
Project Manager: *Camilla Rockwood*
Illustration Manager: *Mick Ruddy*
Designer: *Andy Chapman*

Active Management of Labour
The Dublin Experience

Fourth edition

Kieran O'Driscoll
Declan Meagher

with Michael Robson

National Maternity Hospital
and University College Dublin

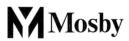 Mosby

Edinburgh London New York Oxford Philadelphia St Louis Sydney Toronto 2003

MOSBY
An affiliate of Elsevier Limited

First edition 1980
Second Edition 1986
Third edition 1993
Fourth edition 2003

ISBN 0 723 43202 3

British Library Cataloguing in Publication Data
A catalogue record for this book is available from the British Library

Library of Congress Cataloging in Publication Data
A catalog record for this book is available from the Library of Congress

Notice
Medical knowledge is constantly changing. Standard safety precautions must be followed, but as new research and clinical experience broaden our knowledge, changes in treatment and drug therapy may become necessary or appropriate. Readers are advised to check the most current product information provided by the manufacturer of each drug to be administered to verify the recommended dose, the method and duration of administration, and contraindications. It is the responsibility of the practitioner, relying on experience and knowledge of the patient, to determine dosages and the best treatment for each individual patient. Neither the Publisher nor the authors assume any liability for any injury and/or damage to persons or property arising from this publication.

Recognition should be given to the fact that hospital guidelines change and that any one time in The National Maternity Hospital may be different to what is found in this book. The guidelines expressed in this book are aimed at midwives and junior doctors, who constitute the main body of the professional workforce. Consultants and Senior Registrars must make independent decisions in the interest of individual patients for whom they are ultimately responsible.
The Publisher

ELSEVIER
SCIENCE
your source for b
journals and mult
in the health scie
www.elsevierhealth.com

The
Publisher's
licy is to use
manufactured
stainable forests

Printed in China

DEDICATED TO THE MIDWIFERY STAFF
IN THE DELIVERY UNIT OF THE
NATIONAL MATERNITY HOSPITAL IN
RECOGNITION OF THEIR UNFAILING
COOPERATION AT ALL TIMES

Contents

Section III: Clinical Data

Preface to the Fourth Edition

It bears repetition to emphasize that the approach to childbirth described in this Fourth Edition arose from the practical experience at the National Maternity Hospital of the original authors of this text and continues to evolve there. The philosophy and principles presented in the First Edition remain just as relevant today; the prevention of prolonged labour with its associated complications will be as important to women in the future as it has been to women in the past.

Over the last 40 years, society's views on childbirth have undergone considerable change. We need to be sensitive to change; nevertheless, adherence to a uniform, disciplined approach, which includes fail-safe procedures, is a fundamental feature of Active Management of Labour. Any departure, if considered appropriate, should always be authorized at a senior level and documented.

The statistical data for the hospital are updated to 2000. The most notable change in practice since the previous edition is a rise in the incidence of caesarean section rate.

We are grateful to Dr Peter Boylan (Master 1991–1997) and Dr Declan Keane (Master 1998– present) for permission to include the most recent figures and also acknowledge their advice together with that of Kathryn MacQuillan (Labour Ward Manager) in the production of this Fourth Edition.

We are also indebted to Professor Patricio Masoli of the University of Valparaiso for his meticulous translation of the Third Edition into a Spanish language version, and for much helpful cross-cultural advice.

Michael Robson
Assistant Master, The National Maternity Hospital, 1991–1994
Consultant Obstetrician
Editor

Kieran O'Driscoll
Master, The National Maternity Hospital,
1963-1969

Declan Meagher
Master, The National Maternity Hospital,
1970-1976

Preface to the Third Edition

The Third Edition of this book continues to be firmly based on personal experience of everyday clinical practice in a large obstetric unit with extensive teaching commitments. The original motivation, which was to enhance the experience of childbirth for mothers with none of the textbook abnormalities, remains substantially unchanged. The format too stays the same. Because the seemingly inexorable rise in caesarean birth rates has come to represent a public health issue of major proportions in many countries, the comparatively low surgical delivery rate maintained in this institution over the years has attracted considerable attention at international level. It seems fitting to emphasise, therefore, that these low surgical delivery rates were not pursued as an end in themselves, but emerged as a reflection of labour management. It is a pleasure to acknowledge our indebtedness to Dr Dermot MacDonald (Master 1977–1983) and Dr Niall O'Brien (Consultant Paediatrician) and to Dr Adrian Grant of the National Perinatal Epidemiology Unit at Oxford, for permission to abstract from what has become generally known as the Dublin Trial of the comparative value of electronic fetal heart monitors, expressed in terms of immediate survival and in terms of cerebral palsy after 4 years of age. This classical study is freely drawn upon in chapters 23 and 28; reference to the complete texts, which are cited in the List of Publications, is strongly recommended. The statistical data for the hospital are updated to 1990; we are grateful to Dr John Stronge (Master 1984–1990) for permission to include the most recent figures.

Kieran O'Driscoll

Declan Meagher

Peter Boylan

Preface to the First Edition

The authors are indebted to very many persons, too numerous to mention, for advice over the years. First, it must be said that a project of this nature could not even have been contemplated without the wholehearted cooperation of the Nursing Sisters in the delivery unit, whose high standards of professional achievement were matched by a flexible attitude to new ideas to a degree that made everything possible. Likewise, our junior medical colleagues, who occupied the position of Assistant Master and whose names have appeared as co-authors of several publications in the medical press: they shared the responsibility for the welfare of every woman and child delivered and made many contributions to the underlying philosophy. And our medical colleagues farther afield, of whom a few only are mentioned here by name, because they made specific recommendations which we have incorporated as standard practice in the management of labour: Dr E.A. Friedman for the graphic representation of cervical dilatation, Dr R.H. Philpott for the introduction of an action-line, and Dr C.H. Hendricks for the suggestions that the duration of labour be measured from the time of admission to a delivery unit. We also wish to acknowledge our debt to the staff of the Physiotherapy Department and to the staff of the Medical Records Department for valuable assistance through the years. Finally, we are grateful to Dr Dermot MacDonald, presently Master of the National Maternity Hospital, for his encouragement in this undertaking.

Kieran O'Driscoll
Master 1963–1969

Declan Meagher
Master 1970–1976

Preface to the First Edition

Introduction

The purpose of this manual is to present the principles, the practice and the results of Active Management of Labour as it has evolved at the National Maternity Hospital over the last 40 years. The contents represent the fruits of the experience of the original authors who, as Masters of the hospital, were responsible for 100 000 births, and of their successors in office, each for a duration of 7 years, which brings the total number of births included to almost 300 000. The text is based on active involvement at every stage of the birth process with meticulous documentation of the outcome in each case; hence the title of the manual. A comprehensive approach to the conduct of labour as practised some 20 times every day, in one of the largest maternity units in Western Europe, is described. This is neither an academic exercise nor a review of medical literature.

The underlying philosophy is firmly based on curtailment of duration of exposure to stress, with avoidance of the physical and emotional trauma, which is likely to follow prolonged labour. With this in mind, efficient uterine action is recognized as the key factor.

The application of this concept requires that a clear distinction be drawn between first and later births, between spontaneous and induced labour, and between singleton cephalic pregnancies and a small number of designated obstetric abnormalities. Malpresentations, malformations and twins are excluded from consideration under the last heading and to these conditions the principles of Active Management of Labour do not apply; together they represent less than 10% of all births.

In practice, a correct initial diagnosis of labour is regarded as a matter of prime importance in every woman admitted to the labour ward. From that point onwards, continuous personal attention on a one-to-one basis is assured at all hours of the day and night. Less apparent is the organizational framework that permits these guidelines to be applied with ease in an exceptional number of cases. Although entirely midwifery based, the labour ward of the National Maternity Hospital benefits from a close working relationship between midwives and obstetricians at every level, leading to a congenial working environment. To complete the picture, each of these items is woven into an overall pattern by rigorous peer review, involving both disciplines, at regular formal sessions.

The contents of this manual are addressed primarily to obstetricians and midwives as the people most directly involved with the provision of care in labour, but are hardly less relevant for anaesthetists, childbirth educators, physiotherapists

1

and, indeed, for others who strive towards this common end. In addition, as no expert knowledge is needed to comprehend the universal significance of the principles enunciated, women themselves will find the text useful, as will medical students and student midwives in contact with the birth process for the first time. Although the principles of Active Management of Labour remain valid in all circumstances, the practice should be considered only in the context of a suitable hospital environment, not in the home.

Background

Although childbirth has long ceased to present a serious physical challenge to healthy women in western society, the emotional impact of labour remains a matter of common concern. In orthodox medical circles, recognition has come slowly that labour, especially first labour, may be the most disturbing emotional event in the lifetime of one-half of humankind. Failure to place enough emphasis on this aspect of the subject is often attributed to the fact that obstetricians are mostly men, although midwives, as women, have shown no greater insight. Rather, the correct explanation seems to us to be that for far too long there has been a tacit acceptance of the conservative, or passive, attitude to labour where nothing could be done to resolve an admittedly unpleasant situation without the introduction of serious extraneous hazards with possible adverse effects on both mother and child. Many would feel that nothing should be done until an impasse is reached. According to this viewpoint, which still gains wide credence, there is no safe alternative to the well-tried doctrine of watchful expectancy and then, if there are any problems, these can readily be solved by operative intervention. Watchful expectancy covers the tedious hours of the first stage of labour, often with the support of drugs or epidural analgesia, until the cervix reaches full dilatation. At this point the outlook tends to change dramatically, so that almost any procedure aimed at early delivery becomes acceptable. This sudden change – from an extremely conservative approach in the first stage to an equally radical approach in the second stage – epitomizes passive management, which is contrary to the philosophy of Active Management of Labour.

As the problem of maternal mortality has receded into history, medical attention has been transferred to the child. Perinatal mortality and, to an increasing degree, perinatal morbidity have become the touchstones of modern obstetrics. One result of this change is that labour, nowadays, is made even more arduous for mothers by the introduction of procedures undertaken in the name of the child, often with scant evidence as to their real value. Somehow the idea seems to have gained ground that a conflict of interest necessarily exists between mother and child during labour and that mothers can be subjected to almost any form of indignity or any degree of discomfort provided this is well intentioned and undertaken on behalf of the child. The philosophy of Active Management of Labour does not subscribe to this proposition: on the contrary, it believes that what is good for mothers is good for babies too, particularly where short duration of labour and delivery without trauma are concerned. A main aim of this manual is to redress the growing imbalance in the birth process to help the mother, without detriment to her child.

The importance of continual audit in Active Management of Labour is paramount. As long ago as 1963 a concerted effort was begun to improve the quality of care extended to all women in labour in the National Maternity Hospital. This hospital was in an exceptionally favourable position to embark on such a project for two main reasons: first, in numerical terms, it was and still is one of the largest maternity units in Western Europe and, second, with the Mastership system, one obstetrician is ultimately responsible for the welfare of all mothers and babies. These inherent advantages afford a unique opportunity to establish a uniform pattern of care in a large number of cases. Finally, there is an efficient system of medical records that is reflected in the timely publication of an Annual Clinical Report with extensive international circulation. A continuous medical audit system ensures that every important aspect of obstetric practice is kept under constant review, so that labour is not considered as a subject in isolation from all other aspects of childbirth, such as caesarean section. The incidence of caesarean section in the National Maternity Hospital has increased sharply in recent years, although the fraction attributed to abnormal labour (dystocia) remains constant.

Meanwhile, in other centres, a growing tendency to resolve the problems of the first stage of labour by surgical intervention has resulted in an alarming increase in the number of caesarean sections attributed to dystocia. Caesarean section rates are currently one of the most realistic objective measures of the standard of obstetric care afforded to mothers, replacing maternal mortality rates, which are outmoded for this purpose in developed countries. By this criterion the overall standard of care afforded to mothers has declined markedly in recent times. Perinatal mortality rates must continue to serve the same purpose in infants until such time as morbidity rates are sufficiently clearly defined.

Procedure

Before any worthwhile improvement in the conduct of labour could even be contemplated, it was evident that the person ultimately responsible must return to the delivery unit to assume direct responsibility for the welfare of all mothers, not just in theory but also in practice. Whereas previously the consultant obstetrician had been involved in only a small number of abnormal cases of eclampsia, breech presentation or diabetes mellitus, who happened to be in labour, they must now become involved directly with the much larger number of perfectly normal women who had hitherto been overlooked at consultant level because they suffered from neither obstetrical complication nor organic disease. Furthermore, it is clear that this commitment must begin at admission and continue until delivery. The consultant, rather than remaining off-stage awaiting the occasional summons to perform an emergency operation in a belated attempt to retrieve a situation which could have been anticipated at a much earlier stage, must seek to prevent such emergencies arising in women who were normal when first admitted

3

to hospital in labour. Ironically, it is in completely normal women that most of the problems of labour arise.

The position of the Sister, or senior midwife in charge of the delivery unit, was seen as a matter of no less importance. Although closely involved at all stages of labour hitherto, she had remained largely powerless to influence the course of events. Apart from the possible administration of analgesic drugs, she lacked clear guidance on how to proceed when storm clouds began to gather. Yet, in spite of this anomaly she was constantly exposed to the possibility of unfair criticism from either side. These genuine grievances have contributed to a generally low state of morale among midwifery staff and remain a serious problem in many delivery units. One of the most important issues raised in this manual is an urgent need to define the professional relationships that should exist between doctors and midwives at different levels of experience. Only when this issue is resolved in a mutually satisfactory manner will it be possible to develop the genuine team spirit which is an essential feature of an efficient service. Adoption of good resolutions to improve the quality of care offered to all women in labour is worthless without the unqualified cooperation of midwifery staff because, in the final analysis, it is midwifery staff who must convert resolutions into practice.

From the outset, the delivery unit in this hospital was designated an intensive care area, wherein every woman and unborn child must be reviewed by a competent medical officer, in the company of the midwife in charge, at regular intervals, especially late at night and early in the morning. The official record of each individual delivered during the previous 24 hours was made the object of special scrutiny by the authors and a current account of the main events was maintained on a daily basis. In this way the consultant obstetrician became actively involved in the conduct of labour on a regular basis as never before; hence the origin of the term 'active management of labour'. The word 'active', in this context, refers to the nature of the involvement of the consultant obstetrician; it certainly is not intended to convey to the reader that they intervene more often. Indeed, precisely the opposite is the case, as the low figures for all forms of operative intervention clearly illustrate. Active participation in the day-to-day functions of the delivery unit by the person ultimately responsible opened entirely new prospects on care in labour; these have led to a fundamental reappraisal of almost all the conventional wisdoms, many of which proved false. Although not apparently based on any factual evidence, these 'wisdoms' had been relayed from teacher to student and textbook to textbook without any serious attempt at verification, until they had come to represent possibly the main impediment to progress in the field.

As a result of this extensive personal and carefully documented experience, care in labour is now based squarely on the simple proposition that efficient uterine action is the key to normality. A strictly pragmatic approach has shown beyond doubt that efficient uterine action can be provided with a very high degree of safety, subject to a small number of rules which are precisely stated. As a consequence of these new-found certainties, a dynamic approach to the birth process, based on efficient uterine action, has replaced the old static approach based largely

4

on pelvic architecture. What may aptly be described as the domino effect of efficient uterine action has left no aspect of labour untouched and, in particular, has brought about a situation in which every expectant mother who attends this hospital for antenatal care is given two firm assurances: that labour will not last longer than 12 hours and that she will not be left without a personal midwife by her side at any time. These two virtual guarantees have changed the face of women's expectations of labour. Taken together, they come close to the kernel of the problem of care in labour while in practice they remain entirely dependent on each other.

Presentation

This manual is divided into three sections.

Section I

The main text consists of a description of the aspects of labour that the authors consider to be of such fundamental importance that each must be examined in considerable detail before any genuine progress can be made. These items are named in the Contents and special notice should be paid to the list of chapter headings because these are topics not often discussed in standard textbooks. No single item can be safely omitted because, like the various pieces of a jigsaw puzzle, they fit snugly together to form a composite picture of which no one fragment can be left out. The language used is both simple and direct. Technical and Latinate terms are purposely avoided because they frequently serve as a cloak that obscures true meaning.

In the opening chapters, particular attention is directed to the absolute need to distinguish clearly between first and all subsequent births, between induction of labour and acceleration of labour that has already started, and to the fact that obstetrical abnormalities – specifically malpresentations, malformation and twins – must always be excluded before consideration can be given to care in labour as a distinct entity. This manual is therefore concerned solely with the prototypal woman in spontaneous labour, i.e. the nulliparous woman with a single cephalic pregnancy. In subsequent chapters the basic parameters of labour are carefully defined, and the rules that govern the use of oxytocin to accelerate progress when labour is slow are stated in quite explicit terms.

In later chapters the causes of abnormal labour are examined, and in the course of this examination the conventional deference shown to cephalopelvic disproportion, which has so dominated attitudes towards labour in former times, is totally rejected. Several chapters are devoted to consideration of the age-old problem of maternal stress, and here the emphasis is on communication as a vital ingredient of good care. Drugs are said to play a minor, but largely unsatisfactory, role.

The closing chapters are concerned with the organization of a busy delivery unit where efficiency and human compassion can coexist. Organization is regarded as a matter of fundamental importance on which all else must ultimately depend. Indeed, poor organization is identified as the rock on which good intentions, in the medical sphere, most often founder. A chapter on induction of labour is included, in the somewhat vain hope that it may serve to dispel at least some of the obfuscation which bedevils this topic; another chapter deals with the relationship between effacement and dilatation of the cervix, since these expressions are in constant use but are seldom accurately defined. There then follows a chapter on caesarean section rates which seem sure to develop into one of the most contentious medical issues of our time. Finally, the tragedy of cerebral palsy, which for various reasons has come to cast a threatening shadow over the whole question of labour management, is examined in the context of the practice set down in these pages.

A few terms may benefit from definition because of different interpretation in other centres: a nulliparous woman is a woman who has not previously given birth to a viable infant; a senior resident requires a specialist qualification in obstetrics and gynaecology; and a resident medical officer is in the process of training.

Section II

The second section consists of a series of visual case records, each selected to illustrate one important aspect of labour, with a brief explanatory note on the facing page. These visual records, or partograms, illustrate better than words ever can the problems that arise in the course of everyday practice. Together they constitute an identikit with which it is possible to construct an endless variety of profiles of labour to meet almost any clinical circumstance. The authors regard this as perhaps the most instructive section of the book because by concentrating the mind it involves the reader directly in the study of labour as a practical, rather than a theoretical, pursuit.

The design and content of these visual records are matters that have an immediate impact on the conduct of labour. The model used in the National Maternity Hospital is worthy of close attention because it is the final product of several years of gradual development in the light of personal experience gained on the floor of a busy delivery unit. Simplicity is the keynote: every detail not immediately relevant to the main issue is rigorously excluded. The graph which portrays progress dominates the picture and no provision is made for labour to last longer than 12 hours. Two colours of partogram distinguish nulliparous from parous women. This is a basic requirement. The point is emphasized repeatedly in the course of the text. A loose-leaf arrangement facilitates retention of all visual records of labour in two clip-in folders: one for nulliparous women and one for parous women. These are retained in the delivery unit where they are available for inspection and discussion. This simple device allows a continuous audit of all the relevant items, which in turn provides a very effective method of central control of the entire service.

The educational potential of these case records is limitless. They have made a unique contribution to the general understanding of the birth process in the National Maternity Hospital and have proved an invaluable aid in the education of both doctors and nurses, and indeed mothers too; mothers perhaps most of all, because they are used as the focus of antenatal preparation for labour. In addition, they continue to provide fertile ground for clinical research and for graduate seminars that can be conducted like exercises in map reading, where mere names become real places as soon as they are located in relation to the surrounding terrain. A serious student can quickly compile a personal series of case records to illustrate the whole gamut of labour experience and in the process construct a storehouse of practical information. Success in this direction is determined by the ability of visual records to speak for themselves and thus reflect a live and durable portrait of one woman and her child in labour.

Section III

The third section consists of a summary of the clinical material that passed through the National Maternity Hospital during the years when Active Management of Labour became standard practice. This information provides the factual background to the text. As events in labour seldom happen in isolation, action taken in one direction is likely to have repercussions in another. Thus, to restrict the duration of labour to 12 hours would serve no useful purpose were this to be achieved at the expense of a significant increase in the incidence of caesarean section in the case of the mother, and mortality or morbidity in the case of the child. The facts will enable readers to see for themselves that statements made in the text are not based on purely theoretical considerations. They also enable comparisons to be made with results from other centres. Best of all, the figures demonstrate the balance that has been struck between one outcome of labour and another. Information of this scope is too often missing from publications that are confined to one narrow aspect of labour; epidural anaesthesia is one of many such examples. Such a form of selective reporting can conceal a significant underlying distortion in the overall picture.

Publications on the subject of labour that emanated from the National Maternity Hospital during the same period are listed elsewhere in this book. These correspond broadly with the chapter headings.

In conclusion, the authors recommend strongly that the pages of this manual be read through consecutively, from beginning to end.

Section I

Nulliparous v Parous Women   1

There are fundamental differences between a first birth and all subsequent births. These differences are so great that they warrant the statement that nulliparous and parous women behave as different biological species. The precise nature of the differences between nulliparous and parous women must be appreciated before care in labour can be established on any semblance of a rational basis.[1]

To ensure that the fundamental differences between a first and a subsequent birth are kept constantly in mind in the National Maternity Hospital, the partogram is printed on paper of two different colours: yellow for nulliparous and blue for parous women. The result is that the first item of information which confronts even the most casual observer is that a woman in labour has, or has not, given birth previously. This remarkably simple device has had a major impact on labour management (see *Partograms 1* and *28*, pp. 135 and 191, respectively).

Unique experience

Modern care in labour, as it relates to the welfare of mothers, is concerned primarily with emotional rather than with physical stress. Labour represents a significant physical challenge to very few women in contemporary practice, and these individuals are generally identified beforehand because they suffer from systemic diseases. The birth of a first child, however, is almost surely the most profound emotional experience, for good or ill, in a lifetime. The first experience of childbirth is of paramount importance because it determines the attitude to all subsequent births.

A woman who has had a happy first experience is unlikely to suffer much apprehension about a later birth, whereas a woman who has had an unhappy first experience is likely to be terrified at the prospect of a repeat performance. These fears can have grave consequences outside the narrow confines of obstetrics; they can haunt a woman for the rest of her life and affect her attitude to her husband and also possibly to her child. Typically, the residual effect of an unhappy first experience is revealed in a second pregnancy by an urgent request for epidural anaesthesia or caesarean section as an opening gambit at the initial antenatal visit, in the firm expectation that the previous ordeal is likely to be repeated. Prompt accession to this request reinforces the fear, for which there is absolutely no foundation in clinical practice. A first labour is unique; the sequence of events that takes place on that occasion has no relevance to later births. The lesson is simple: provide a high standard of care and attention first time round and a woman will require little assistance on the next occasion. Conversely, the damage inflicted by a low standard of care and attention in a first labour is usually irreversible.

Prolonged labour

The most distinctive feature of first labour is duration. A first labour is longer because inefficient uterine action is common and because the genital tract has not previously been stretched. This applies equally to the cervix in the first stage and to the vagina in the second stage. Slow progress in a nulliparous woman should always be regarded as an expression of inefficient uterine action; the possibility of cephalopelvic disproportion should not even be entertained until efficient uterine action has been assured.

The duration of a subsequent labour is comparatively short, partly because inefficient uterine action is a rare occurrence in parous women, and partly because the genital tract has been stretched on a previous occasion. Slow progress in labour in a parous woman should never be assumed to be an expression of inefficient uterine action, but rather an expression of obstruction caused by a fetal complication, such as malpresentation or malformation. This obstruction can easily lead to rupture of uterus in a parous woman, especially if oxytocin is used to expedite delivery.

Cephalopelvic disproportion

Another distinctive feature of first labour is cephalopelvic disproportion. This possibility arises simply because the functional capacity of the pelvis is not yet known. The term 'cephalopelvic disproportion' should be restricted to nulliparous women to avoid confusion with obstructed labour in parous women in whom the functional capacity of the pelvis is already proven. Obstructed labour in a parous woman is a different clinical entity altogether and is fraught with far more sinister consequences for both mother and child. Cephalopelvic disproportion is linked erroneously in the collective subconscious of obstetricians with fear of serious injury to mother and child. This mistaken association of ideas has greatly impeded improvements in the supervision of labour for many years.

Rupture of uterus

Another distinctive feature of first labour is immunity to rupture. Rupture of the uterus is such an exceptional event in nulliparous women that for practical purposes it can be assumed not to occur, except as a result of manipulation. Nulliparous women do not cause injury to themselves or to their children. Serious injury to a nulliparous woman, of which rupture of uterus is the ultimate example, is inflicted, usually with instruments. This is one of the most important clinical observations in the entire field of obstetrics. In particular, this observation has led us to a complete reappraisal of the hitherto general assumption that oxytocin may cause rupture of uterus in the presence of undetected cephalopelvic disproportion. There is now ample evidence that this assumption, which has dominated the supervision of labour for so long, has no foundation in practice. There can be no doubt whatsoever that the mistake arose from failure to draw a sufficiently clear distinction between nulliparous and parous women in labour. Indeed, the fear that oxytocin may cause rupture of the uterus is only too well founded in parous women: whereas nulliparous women are rupture proof, parous women are rupture prone. The inherent tendency of the parous uterus to rupture is a factor that must be taken into account whenever the potential risks of epidural anaesthesia are under consideration.

Traumatic intracranial haemorrhage

Yet another distinctive feature of first labour is the likelihood of serious injury to the child. Rupture of tentorium cerebelli, with consequent subdural haemorrhage, is the extreme example. This lesion corresponds with rupture of uterus in the mother. Rupture of tentorium occurs during the second stage of labour and, in cephalic presentation, is almost invariably associated with instrumental delivery. Consequently, serious injury to the child occurs much more often in nulliparous women; not because of cephalopelvic disproportion but because of the comparatively high incidence of forceps delivery. The influence of epidural anaesthesia is relevant in this context.

Extensive experience with oxytocin to ensure efficient uterine action in nulliparous women has shown that the risk of serious injury to both mother and child has been reduced because the need for vaginal operative delivery has fallen. Risk of birth injury declines when babies are born by propulsion rather than by traction. Trauma is discussed as a separate item in Chapter 14 (see also *Tables 4* and *5*, pp. 201 and 203, respectively).

Key Points

- Nulliparous and parous women should be considered separately in labour
- Inefficient uterine action is the most common complication of labour in nulliparous women; it is rare in parous women
- The nulliparous uterus is virtually immune to rupture, whereas the parous uterus is rupture prone
- Provide a high standard of care in the first labour and the woman will require little assistance on the next occasion

Induction v Acceleration

2

Just as there are fundamental differences between a first and a subsequent birth, there are fundamental differences between induction and acceleration. There exists a quite remarkable degree of confusion between these two procedures, despite the fact that a clear appreciation of the essential differences is a prerequisite to a rational approach to care in labour.

Failure to make a sufficiently sharp distinction between an attempt to interrupt the natural course of pregnancy on the one hand, and to accelerate the course of labour – as a physiological process which has already begun – on the other, has misled doctors, nurses and mothers into the vague assumption that induction and acceleration are somehow extensions of the same procedure, merging imperceptibly into each other. This confusion stems mainly from the fact that membranes are ruptured artificially and oxytocin is infused in both instances. The logic of this position is comparable to a conclusion that no distinction need be drawn between diseases so totally dissimilar as amoebic dysentery and trichomonal vaginitis, because the therapeutic agent is identical.

Duration of stress

Induction has the opposite effect to acceleration because induction extends the period of stress to which a woman is exposed – by the length of time that elapses before labour begins. As the main purpose of acceleration is to limit the period of stress to which a woman in labour is exposed, there is an obvious need to examine very closely indeed all aspects of a procedure that has precisely the opposite result.

Diagnosis of labour

The diagnosis of labour is often hopelessly obfuscated by induction. This is because artificial rupture of membranes is performed as part of the procedure and painful uterine contractions are stimulated with oxytocin. Even in normal circumstances painful uterine contractions are not reliable evidence of labour, but when they occur in response to oxytocin, they must be regarded with even greater suspicion. Pains caused by oxytocin are very likely to cease should the infusion be withdrawn. Therefore, it is a mistake to base a diagnosis of labour on evidence of painful uterine contractions, supported by a 'show' or ruptured membranes, as recommended in spontaneous labour. Pains caused by prostaglandins may be equally misleading. The diagnosis of labour in a case of induction must rest on dilatation of cervix alone. The result is that it is well-nigh impossible to state at which point in time, if indeed ever, induction ends and labour begins. The critical importance of a correct initial diagnosis in the supervision of labour is discussed at some length in Chapter 5 where it is stated that diagnosis is the single most important issue in the care of labour and, furthermore, that whenever the diagnosis is wrong every action which follows is likely to compound the error. Nowhere is this more clearly apparent than in cases of induction.

Operative intervention

There is a sharp increase in the rate of surgical intervention in cases of induction. However, caesarean sections performed after induction are more often than not attributed to complications of labour, such as inefficient uterine action, cephalo-pelvic disproportion or occipitoposterior position, when the reality is that labour has not even started. The explanation is to be found in the mistaken belief that labour begins when a woman on oxytocin complains of painful uterine contractions. Alternatively, caesarean sections performed after induction are attributed to the indications for which the inductions were undertaken, such as pre-eclampsia or prolonged pregnancy, although these indications may seldom bear close scrutiny and would rarely, of themselves, justify caesarean section. There is a natural reluctance to acknowledge the plain truth: that caesarean section after induction is required to retrieve a situation which stems from medical intervention, especially when the indication for this intervention lacks genuine substance.

Favourable comparisons are sometimes made between caesarean section rates in cases in which labour is induced and in cases in which labour is not induced. Such comparisons are false and misleading because they do not compare like with like. Whereas elective caesarean sections are included amongst cases not induced, a decision to induce labour is taken in the expectation of vaginal delivery. It follows that the caesarean section rate in induced cases should be considerably lower than in cases not induced; any discrepancy should be attributed to the procedure itself and separately recorded under the title 'failed induction'.

The vaginal operative delivery rate is also higher following induction. In addition, it is carried out earlier after full dilatation has been achieved because of the extended period of stress to which the woman has been exposed, and for this reason rotation is more likely to be required. Acceleration of labour, by way of contrast, reduces the rate of operative intervention because, labours being shorter, mothers are more likely to effect spontaneous delivery.

Analgesia

There is a sharp increase in demand for pain relief in cases of induction. This is reflected in the dosage of drugs used and in the number of epidurals requested.

The increase in demand for analgesia is a measure of the increase in intensity and duration of stress imposed. A surfeit of drugs introduces further extraneous problems which are discussed in later chapters. Acceleration of labour, on the other hand, reduces demand for analgesia because labour has already begun before the need arises and because steps are then taken to ensure that delivery occurs within a reasonable timescale.

Effects on others

A high rate of induction subjects not only those mothers who are involved directly to a period of stress that is prolonged artificially; the adverse effects extend to encompass all women in labour. A high rate of induction has an important indirect bearing on others because the limited resources of a delivery unit – especially the human resources – are dissipated in caring for women who are not in labour. This dilution of personal attention, which is a cornerstone of good care, affects everyone; it is at complete variance with the concept of intensive care. It seems a strange paradox of contemporary delivery unit practice that women who are not in labour should receive more attention, and for a longer time, than women who are in labour.

Time and place

To ensure that the sharp distinction between induction and acceleration is continually reinforced, induction is undertaken as an elective procedure at a fixed time of day. Moreover, artificial rupture of membranes to induce labour is not performed in the labour ward. Induction with prostaglandin is performed on the antenatal ward.

Time and place are thus used to reinforce the message. This ensures that clear decisions are made, especially in respect of diagnosis of labour, before any form of intervention is allowed. The rationale is comparable to the use of coloured partograms to differentiate between nulliparous and parous women, as described in Chapter 1. Acceleration of labour and induction of labour are discussed as separate issues in Chapters 8 and 24.

Key Points

- A distinction between spontaneous and induced labour must be rigidly maintained
- Induction has numerous adverse effects on the outcome of labour

Malpresentations, Malformation, Twins   **3**

The third fundamental distinction which must be drawn before labour can be discussed in a rational manner is between care in labour and treatment of obstetrical abnormalities. The present treatise, on care in labour, is confined to cases in which there is a single fetus, a vertex presentation and a normal head. Obstetrical abnormalities, particularly those which implicate the fetus directly, are specifically excluded from consideration because, inter alia, these may cause obstruction during labour, thus placing the fetus and sometimes even the mother at risk. Treatment of obstetrical abnormalities, which include malpresentations, malformation and twins, is discussed at length in standard textbooks. These topics are as much outside the scope of the present treatise as are obstetrical abnormalities which affect the mother more directly, for example eclampsia or haemorrhage.

A brief outline of the general approach to treatment of malpresentations, relevant malformation and twins is given in this chapter. All subsequent chapters are written on the clear assumption that definitive steps have been taken to exclude these conditions beforehand. Nonetheless, all admissions are included in the final statistics.

Breech and face

The hazards of breech delivery are confined to the child; virtually the only danger to the mother is through obstetrical intervention. The approach to the treatment of breech presentation in labour is pragmatic. Vaginal delivery has a place whenever this can be accomplished without any form of obstetrical intervention. Caesarean section is the only treatment allowed, whether the need should arise during the first or the second stage of labour. Oxytocin is not used to accelerate slow progress in breech presentation. X-ray pelvimetry is not practised because size and shape of pelvis are not factors taken into account in deciding the mode of delivery.

The approach to face presentation in labour is along similar lines. Vaginal delivery is preferred whenever this can be accomplished without any form of obstetrical intervention. Caesarean section is the only treatment allowed. Oxytocin is not used to accelerate slow progress in face presentation.

Brow and shoulder

Brow presentation and shoulder presentation in labour – the latter a rare occurrence in nulliparous women – are always treated by caesarean section. These are two of the most notable causes of obstructed labour, which can so easily lead to rupture of uterus in parous women. Hence, brow presentation and shoulder presentation differ from breech presentation and face presentation in that they also place the life of the mother at risk. Treatment of malpresentations by corrective manipulation is not practised. Oxytocin is not used.

Hydrocephalus

The only malformation likely to cause obstruction is hydrocephalus. This is the third notable cause of obstructed labour which is likely to lead to rupture of uterus in parous women. The condition is treated on an individual basis according to the circumstances.

Twins

Twins are regarded as an obstetrical abnormality, mainly because the second twin is exposed to the special hazards of hypoxia and, after delivery of the first twin, malpresentation. Administration of oxytocin to twins is highly selective and prescribed only after review by the senior resident on duty.

Obstruction

Notwithstanding the fact that detection of malpresentations, relevant malformation and twins is an integral part of antenatal care, and that independent assessment at the point of admission is also mandatory, the final responsibility rests squarely on the person who makes the decision to use oxytocin to ensure that these obstetrical abnormalities have been excluded in each case. The person who prescribes oxytocin for a woman in labour should be required to place the following items on permanent record: the vertex presents, the head is normal, there is a single fetus. However, in practice, it is in parous women only that malpresentation and malformation present a serious threat to the mother, because it is in parous women only that obstruction is likely to lead to rupture of uterus, whether or not oxytocin is mistakenly used. The reason why oxytocin should be used with extreme caution in parous women, is that the parous uterus is highly vulnerable in this regard. This is certainly not true in nulliparous women. Inadvertently, over time, oxytocin has been given, mistakenly, to nulliparous women with obstructed labour, caused by malpresentation and malformation, but without untoward effect.

The three classic components of abnormal labour – inefficient uterine action, occipitoposterior position and cephalopelvic disproportion – are not classified as obstetrical abnormalities. These are complications of labour which arise in normal cases after admission to hospital. This is a point of great practical importance because there is a belief that cephalopelvic disproportion is an obstetrical abnormality which can be detected before labour begins. This results in many elective caesarean sections which are quite unnecessary and which, moreover, are wrongly reported as examples of cephalopelvic disproportion.

Key Points

- Discussions on labour should be strictly confined to cases where the vertex presents, the head is normal, there is a single fetus and the onset is spontaneous

- Obstetrical abnormalities should be considered separately

Duration of Labour 4

It would be difficult to exaggerate the beneficial effects of an accurate working definition of duration of labour on everyday practice, since failure to define what is clearly one of the basic parameters of clinical obstetrics has been a major obstacle to improvements in management for many years.[2]

Definition

In the National Maternity Hospital, duration of labour is defined as the number of hours a woman spends in the delivery unit from the time of admission until the time her baby is born (see *Figure 4.1*). No allowance is made for time spent in labour at home. Speculation on the number of hours a woman may have been in labour before she chose to admit herself to hospital is a futile exercise. This is an issue which cannot be resolved satisfactorily and which, in any event, has no relevance to subsequent care. Incidentally, the third stage of labour is not included in this definition.

There are four reasons why duration of labour is so defined:

- Time of admission is a maternal decision.
- Professional responsibility begins when a woman elects to place herself in care.
- Duration can be recorded accurately for purposes of comparison.
- Mothers themselves tend to recall duration of labour in this manner.

Effectively, overall duration of labour is determined by the length of the first stage, because the number of hours taken for the cervix to dilate represents some 90% of the entire birth process. The second stage is short by comparison, and contributes little to the problem of prolonged labour.

This definition of duration applies equally when a woman who is not in labour remains in the delivery unit for whatever reason. Hence, duration of labour in the case of a woman admitted for induction is likewise recorded as hours spent in the delivery unit, because this is the actual duration of stress to which she is exposed. Although it is not possible to say at what point induction ends and labour begins, the procedure itself exposes the woman to the same pressures as if she were in labour for all of the time. The definition still applies even when induction fails and resort is made to caesarean section. Similarly, when a woman is retained in the delivery unit in error because of a wrong diagnosis of labour, duration is nonetheless recorded from the time of admission. This means that duration of labour is entered for some women who are recognized in retrospect as not having been in labour at all. Such anomalies demonstrate the extent to which duration of labour is synonymous with time spent in the delivery unit of this hospital.

Advantages of short labour

The mean duration of first labour – without any form of intervention – is 6 hours. In general, women tolerate stress of this duration very well, and provided they have a reasonable understanding of the birth process and are not left alone, they usually succeed in delivering themselves.

To the mother

The impact of labour must be evaluated as much in emotional as in physical terms. Both are more closely related to the number of hours spent in a delivery unit than to any other objective measurement. Although some women are already unduly perturbed at the point of admission, and others remain apparently unmoved after many hours have passed, most fall somewhere between the two extremes. The morale of the average woman begins to deteriorate perceptibly after 6 hours. After 12 hours the deterioration accelerates rapidly – in geometric rather than arithmetic progression – until, eventually, a stage is reached at which an adult woman is reduced to pleading for deliverance, unless she is rendered semi-conscious with drugs or lulled into a false sense of security with epidural anaesthesia. It cannot be emphasized too strongly that the profound emotional disturbance caused by prolonged labour may endure a lifetime. Consequently, no woman should be permitted to continue long enough in labour to need more than two standard doses of analgesia, by whatever route.

Exogenous influences, other than time, which have a significant bearing on the emotional equilibrium of women in labour are: good antenatal education, continuous personal attention, and constructive use of drugs to relieve discomfort. These items are discussed in later chapters.

To the enormously important, if somewhat less tangible, emotional benefits must be added the physical benefits of short labour. Nowadays, no one should be permitted to continue nearly long enough in labour to require treatment for dehydration, ketosis or salt depletion. There is virtually no possibility of these disturbances arising within a strict timescale of 12 hours. These considerations assume even greater relevance in tropical climates where changes of this nature can occur much more rapidly. There are also the noteworthy advantages of a lesser need for surgical intervention (caesarean section during the first stage and rotational forceps during the second stage), simply because mothers are better able to deliver themselves if they are not exhausted. Lastly, there is a greatly reduced demand for analgesic drugs, which means that mothers who are fully conscious remain in complete control.

To the child

Duration of labour is equally important for the child. A fetus is exposed to the risk of hypoxia, mainly in the first stage, and of trauma, mainly in the second stage. There is especially close correlation between trauma and duration because long labours frequently end in difficult vaginal or abdominal operative deliveries. In times past, the medical approach to prolonged labour was based on full dilatation of cervix as the natural line of demarcation between abdominal and vaginal delivery. The primary aim was to sustain the mother and, through her, hopefully, the baby, until full dilatation was reached. Full dilatation became an end in itself, and when this milestone was achieved, the ordeal was brought to a speedy, and often forcible, conclusion. This meant that ventouse or forceps were applied before the head could descend to the level at which rotation into the anterior position naturally occurs. Not infrequently, serious trauma was inflicted in the process. The circle of confusion was complete when the difficult manoeuvre and consequent trauma were interpreted as evidence that prolonged labour, or dystocia, is a common expression of cephalopelvic disproportion. Emphatically, this is not so.

To the staff

Duration of labour is a matter that affects professional staff hardly less profoundly. A shared sense of impotence in the face of widespread physical suffering, and even moral degradation, frequently colours the attitude of nurses and doctors from their early student days. Those who subsequently choose to specialize react in different ways: obstetricians tend to avoid the delivery unit as much as possible, while midwives tend to resort to excessive use of analgesia to alleviate otherwise intolerable personal stress. Control of duration of labour is almost as important for staff as it is for mothers and babies.

To the administrators

Duration of labour is also a matter of utmost practical importance to administrators because the delivery unit constitutes the bottleneck in a maternity service through which all women must pass. The result is that it is not possible to plan maternity hospital accommodation, or to allocate professional staff on a rational basis, unless the total number of hours women are in labour can be calculated in advance. This is an excellent example of the application of principles of cost efficiency in healthcare planning, where good medicine and sound economics complement each other. Nowhere is this seen to better advantage than in a modern and efficient delivery unit.

Conclusion

In the National Maternity Hospital, prolonged labour was defined as 36 hours in 1963, reduced to 24 hours in 1968 and, finally, to 12 hours in 1972. A formal decision was taken on 1 January 1972 to restrict the duration of labour to 12 hours. After that date, no provision was made on the official record for labour to last a longer time. The result is a well-established philosophy, of which all expectant mothers are made fully aware: not to expose anyone to the stress of labour for more than 12 hours. Meanwhile, almost 300 000 babies have been born and every mother not close to an easy vaginal delivery after 12 hours has been delivered by caesarean section. Contrary to reasonable expectations, this practice did not lead to any significant increase in the incidence of caesarean section; what appeared likely to be lost on the swings has been more than recovered on the roundabouts. The wider implications of the relatively lower incidence of caesarean section for dystocia as compared to the startling increase in most other centres over the same period are considered in Chapter 27.

Key Points

- An accurate working definition for duration of labour has significant benefits in everyday practice
- Duration of labour determines the impact of childbirth on mothers, babies and attendants
- Prolonged labour is essentially a problem of first birth

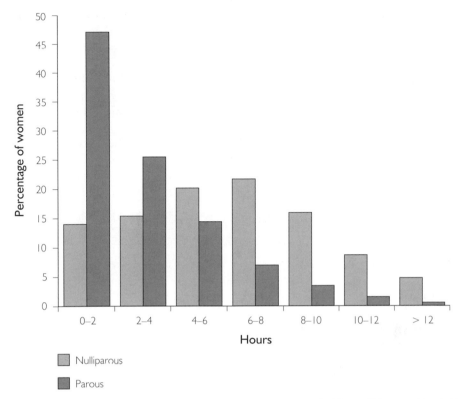

Figure 4.1. Duration of labour from time of admission to delivery unit in the National Maternity Hospital in 2001.

Diagnosis of Labour   5

The most important single issue of care in labour is diagnosis. When the initial diagnosis is wrong, all subsequent care is likely to be also wrong. The unfortunate consequences are to be seen almost daily in our delivery units, although these are seldom recognized for what they are. There is an almost universal failure to appreciate that the diagnosis of labour represents a genuine problem. This has led to the altogether anomalous situation in which the fundamental decision, on which all subsequent care is based, is left to mothers. Uniquely, an expectant mother admits herself to a maternity hospital, with the result that she tends to dictate her own treatment. This method of procedure, which leaves the initiative in the hands of 'patients', has no parallel in other branches of medicine.[3]

Midwives and doctors are noticeably vague whenever questions are asked about diagnosis of labour. Hence it should come as no surprise that mothers, especially nulliparous women who lack previous experience, should sometimes be mistaken and admit themselves to hospital in error. Perhaps the most surprising feature is not that mothers are sometimes wrong, but that they are usually right. There are very few maternity centres where any serious attention is devoted to the diagnosis of labour. The general assumption is that no such problem exists, because women are naturally endowed with an unerring instinct that enables them to make a correct decision in these matters. The subject is not discussed at any length in textbooks and is evaded in medical publications, where only cases said to be in 'established' labour – because the cervix is well dilated – are included in scientific reports. Common practice is to resort to the convenient device of making a retrospective decision that a woman has been in labour after her baby is born. In everyday practice, however, decisions must be prospective; real life does not afford the luxury of wisdom after the event. An essential difference between the theory and the practice of care in labour is that the midwife does not enjoy the benefit of hindsight when an agitated nulliparous woman presents herself at a delivery unit late at night because she thinks she is in labour. A firm decision is required in these circumstances. Equivocal terms such as 'false labour', 'latent labour' or 'labour not established' serve only as stratagems to relieve the attendant of the onus of having to make this decision. Such terms have no real meaning. The effect, however, is to pass the responsibility for the diagnosis of labour back to the woman, where it certainly does not belong. Most errors in the care of labour result from decisions avoided, rather than from decisions wrongly made. This dictum applies with particular force to the initial diagnosis.

First step

The first step in the care of labour is to confirm, or deny, the presumptive diagnosis that has been made by the mother prior to admission. There are strict instructions to this effect and these instructions must be put into practice no later than 1 hour after admission. The midwife in charge of the delivery unit is nominated as the person directly responsible. The official chart, or partogram, is designed in such a manner as to ensure that the evidence on which her decision is based is committed to permanent record. The terms are both simple and explicit. This evidence is located in the most prominent position. Thus, a prospective diagnosis of labour is made in every case admitted and the evidence on which this was based remains available, even when the individual concerned has gone off duty (see *Partogram 3*, p. 139).

Meanwhile, no procedure whatsoever is permitted until a firm diagnosis of labour is made, because of the concern of committing a woman to delivery when she is not in labour. Naturally, whenever a woman's presumptive diagnosis of labour is not accepted by staff she deserves an adequate explanation, couched in simple language that she can understand. The explanation given is a paraphrase of what is written here; it is almost universally well received. Attendance at antenatal classes would have prepared the woman for this eventuality. The woman is then transferred to the antenatal ward where she is retained until the next day. A woman who is adjudged not to be in labour is not retained in the delivery unit for one moment longer than is absolutely necessary and never for longer than 1 hour.

Pains

A woman's diagnosis of labour is based on the subjective element of pain. Pain is such a constant feature that without pain the question of labour simply does not arise. However, not every woman who complains of pain is necessarily in labour, although late in pregnancy this is by no means an unreasonable assumption. The nature and distribution of the particular pain may be so uncharacteristic that it bears no resemblance whatever to labour, in which case it can be discounted readily by an experienced observer. Alternatively, the pain may be so characteristic – intermittent, symmetrical and coincident with uterine contractions – that it can make for a much more difficult decision.

There is a popular misconception, prevalent even in professional circles, that pain which coincides with uterine contractions provides conclusive evidence of labour. This is an elementary mistake. A doctor or midwife with hand on abdomen to confirm that a woman winces as her uterus contracts needs to appreciate that Braxton Hicks contractions, which are a normal feature of late pregnancy, increase both in strength and frequency as term approaches and, furthermore, that they can cause considerable discomfort when the threshold for pain is low. Pain of this nature cannot be distinguished from pain of labour because of the common origin. The threshold for pain is reduced mainly through anxiety, which is most likely to occur late at night, especially when a woman is alone, or resides at a considerable distance from the hospital service. Understandably, a woman who fears that she may arrive too late tends to travel too early. These are salient factors that should be taken into account when a diagnosis of labour is under consideration.

An air of uncertainty at the point of admission compounds the problem still further, because the woman quickly senses that the experts from whom she had a right to expect guidance cannot even recognize labour! Instead of firm direction she meets with evasion, which undermines her confidence even more. As anxiety increases the pain worsens. Unfortunately, staff are wont to respond with analgesic drugs; these have the indirect effect of committing the woman to delivery. Therefore, it must be made crystal clear that painful uterine contractions alone do not warrant a professional diagnosis of labour. Painful uterine contractions need to be supported by evidence of a more objective nature before a professional diagnosis of labour can be upheld.

Effacement and dilatation

Diagnosis of labour presents no problem whenever painful uterine contractions are combined with dilatation of cervix, since the very essence of labour is the opening of the neck of the womb. A woman who enters hospital with her cervix well dilated is not only surely in labour, but also can be expected to progress rapidly and deliver normally within a matter of a few hours. The extent of dilatation of the cervix at the point of admission is a clear indication of the efficiency of uterine action: it is not, as often supposed, a reflection of the number of hours spent in labour at home. Reports in the literature, which are confined to cases in which labour is said to be 'established', do not merely evade the fundamental problem of diagnosis, they also exclude from consideration the very cases that are likely to cause problems in subsequent care. As these are the women who suffer from inefficient uterine action, such selective reporting can be very misleading.

Since dilatation of cervix represents the sole conclusive evidence of labour, it is clearly essential that this term be accurately defined. Of necessity, this entails definition of the term effacement also, because the two events are closely related and frequently confused. Chapter 26 is devoted to consideration of these two critical events in greater detail. Meanwhile, the term 'effacement' refers to incorporation of the cervical canal into the lower uterine segment. This proceeds from above downwards, i.e. from the internal os to the external os. The process may either occur late in pregnancy or be delayed until labour begins. Dilatation, on the other hand, refers only to the external os. This does not begin to open until the entire length of the canal has been eliminated, at which point effacement is complete. As this marks a point of transition, to speak of dilatation before effacement is complete involves a direct contradiction of terms.

The external os is seldom so tightly closed that it does not admit a fingertip long before labour is due to begin. This can be a source of confusion when a fingertip is equated with 1 cm on the notional metric scale used to express the extent of dilatation of cervix during labour. Effacement is the feature that serves to distinguish between the cervix that passively admits a fingertip and the cervix that is dilated to the extent of 1 cm in labour. A diagnosis of labour is made when a woman admits herself with painful uterine contractions and the cervix is found to be completely effaced on pelvic examination. Such a woman is retained in the delivery unit and therefore committed to delivery within 12 hours.

With regard to diagnosis of labour, the problem cases are to be found among the considerable number of women who admit themselves to hospital with painful uterine contractions but in whom the cervix is not completely effaced. In these circumstances, objective evidence of a different order must be sought, in particular a 'show' or spontaneous rupture of membranes. These simple signs provide invaluable aids to diagnosis when the cervix is not completely effaced.

'Show'

A 'show', or bloodstained plug of mucus, passed early – often before effacement is complete and dilatation can begin – is easily recognized by both mothers and staff and, consequently, has an important role to play in the diagnosis of labour. Although not conclusive, a show affords presumptive evidence of dynamic change in the condition of the cervix which is sufficient to cause the plug of mucus to be extruded.

A diagnosis of labour is made when subjective evidence of pain is supported by objective evidence of a show, even though the cervix may not be totally effaced, let alone dilated. A woman with painful uterine contractions and a show is retained in the delivery unit and consequently, committed to delivery, without regard to the condition of the cervix. An exception is sometimes made in the case of a woman who is less than 37 weeks' gestation, in the somewhat vain hope that labour may be somehow averted. A show has already occurred in approximately 70% of women who admit themselves to the National Maternity Hospital in the belief that they are in labour.

Naturally, a show without painful uterine contractions does not warrant the same interpretation. A show in such circumstances is recorded as an unsubstantial antepartum haemorrhage, and the woman is transferred to the antenatal ward. A show which follows vaginal examination is regarded as an artefact, about which anyone undergoing the procedure is given a prior explanation.

Ruptured membranes

Spontaneous rupture of membranes is accepted as even stronger presumptive evidence of labour than a show. A diagnosis of labour is made when a woman admits herself with painful uterine contractions supported by spontaneous rupture of membranes. She is retained in the delivery unit and, therefore, committed to delivery within 12 hours, even if the cervix is only partially effaced. Spontaneous rupture of membranes has already occurred in approximately 30% of women who admit themselves to the National Maternity Hospital in the belief that they are in labour.

Similarly, spontaneous rupture of membranes alone does not warrant a diagnosis of labour. Membranes not infrequently rupture several weeks before labour eventually begins. A woman with spontaneous rupture of membranes but no painful uterine contractions is transferred to the antenatal ward. A pelvic examination is not performed if there is a likelihood that a woman admitted with spontaneous rupture of the membranes may not be in labour. Induction is performed as an elective procedure. This serves to maintain the sharp distinction between acceleration of labour which has already begun and initiation of labour which has not yet started. Hence, the challenge of diagnosis of labour must be confronted at every step along the way. In the event of a woman with spontaneous rupture of membranes returning to the delivery unit within a few hours, it is not always concluded that the initial decision was necessarily wrong. More likely, the correct explanation in this situation is that meanwhile the woman has, so to speak, induced labour on herself. Rupture of membranes, whether artificial or spontaneous, is an effective method of initiating labour.

A show and spontaneous rupture of membranes count as two independent signs of labour when the show appears first, but as one sign only when the membranes rupture first, because the significance of a show is vitiated by prior rupture of membranes.

Errors in diagnosis

An error in diagnosis of labour can be made either way.

A woman's diagnosis of labour may be accepted, in which case she is retained in the delivery unit and exposed to the manifold pressures of that particular environment. Inevitably, her morale begins to crumble and her physical condition eventually deteriorates as time passes and no progress is made. The problem is compounded by the administration of analgesic drugs or epidural block, and possibly oxytocin, until a point is reached at which there is no option but to terminate her ordeal by resort to caesarean section. The record will doubtless show that caesarean section was performed for maternal or fetal distress caused by prolonged labour, whereas the truth of the matter is that the initial diagnosis of labour was incorrect: a state of labour never existed. The first occasion when such a woman is seen by the consultant obstetrician may well be when the operation is about to be performed. The clinical history available at this juncture is likely, at best, to be second hand. It is also frequently impossible to identify the person who made the critical decision, much less review the evidence on which that decision was based. In practice these questions are seldom even asked, simply because their significance is not widely appreciated.

Alternatively, a woman's diagnosis of labour may be rejected by staff, in which case she is transferred to the antenatal ward, perhaps to return a short time later well advanced in labour. This is not a serious mistake.

A woman's diagnosis of labour is rejected in some delivery units merely because the cervix is only 1 cm dilated, and the woman is not considered to be in 'established labour'. If the diagnosis is delayed, some uteri may fail to respond later to oxytocin, if required.

Of course, it must be acknowledged that no matter how much careful attention is paid to the diagnosis of labour, subsequent events will sometimes prove it wrong, because it is just not possible to make a correct decision in every case. No method of diagnosis is foolproof. The aim should be to reduce the number of errors to a minimum.

The ability to retrieve an admittedly difficult situation depends partly on the sense of trust which the mother places in the staff and partly on the confidence that the staff have in themselves; self-confidence and mutual respect permit mistakes to be acknowledged and freely discussed. These characteristics are very closely related to overall standards of practice in a delivery unit. However, some mothers become so distressed by the unfortunate experience that it is not possible to return to the original position: in this event, caesarean section is the only solution. Nevertheless, the fact remains that the true state of affairs is seldom recognized. Approximately 30% of women who admit themselves under the impression that they are in labour are mistaken. It is a matter of utmost importance that these individuals be identified before they find themselves on a path from which there is but one escape route – caesarean section – and that after much anguish.

Diagnosis after induction

Finally, a note about induction. Anyone who is genuinely concerned about the quality of care in labour must look very closely indeed at the practice of induction, a subject about which more is written in Chapter 24. In the present context, it cannot be emphasized too strongly that a procedure which includes artificial rupture of membranes and infusion of oxytocin plays havoc with the diagnosis of labour. Oxytocin causes painful uterine contractions, whether or not a woman is in labour; this is a vivid example of the commonplace fallacy of basing a diagnosis of labour on painful uterine contractions alone. In the course of induction the significance of painful uterine contractions, a show and ruptured membranes are all nullified. Hence the diagnosis of labour in a case of induction rests solely on dilatation of cervix. The fact that this is not generally appreciated leads to widespread confusion about when induction ends and labour begins. This provides the opportunity of attributing an adverse outcome in such cases to a complication of labour rather than to a failed induction which would be more correct.

There is one other aspect of the problem of diagnosis of labour worthy of brief comment. This concerns claims made for treatment aimed at arresting the course of labour which has started prematurely. The credibility of these claims rests entirely on whether or not the subjects treated were actually in labour to begin with, i.e. on the accuracy of the initial diagnosis. Advocates of this form of therapy tend to start from the premise that the diagnosis of labour is such a simple matter that it can be taken for granted. Needless to say, this is far from the truth. Such scant attention is paid to the problem of diagnosis of labour at term that it may come as a surprise to find the ease with which it is made before term in publications advocating the benefits of tocolytic agents.[4]

Key Points

- Diagnosis is the single most important issue in the supervision of labour
- Diagnosis must be prospective and, in effect, be a positive decision to commit a woman to delivery within 12 hours
- Most errors of care in labour result from decisions avoided rather than decisions wrongly made
- The midwife is responsible for the diagnosis of labour
- Few maternity units pay adequate attention to diagnosis of labour
- The evidence for diagnosis of labour must be placed on permanent record and the outcomes discussed

Progress: First Stage   6

After the diagnosis of labour has been confirmed, the next important item is to monitor progress, at short and regular intervals, especially in the early hours. Progress during the first stage of labour is measured exclusively in terms of dilatation of cervix, because the sole function of uterine action during the first stage of labour is to dilate the cervix to allow the baby's head to pass. The rate of dilatation of cervix is crucial because the duration of labour depends almost entirely on the duration of the first stage. This is true to the extent that the two are almost synonymous in clinical practice. The first stage accounts for some 90% of the entire birth process in normal circumstances.

Descent of head is not an appropriate measure of progress during the first stage of labour. There is no consistent relationship between dilatation of cervix and descent of head. Descent of head is the measure of progress appropriate to the second stage of labour. The sole function of uterine action during the second stage is to propel the fetus along the birth canal.

Pelvic examination

Pelvic examination is performed at the time of admission, and repeated two hours later. Subsequent examinations are performed at intervals, depending on the circumstances. Successive examinations are performed by the same person because there is a considerable subjective element in interpretation. Dilatation of cervix is not susceptible to accurate measurement; consequently, this is one clinical situation where too many cooks will surely spoil the broth. The midwife in charge of the delivery unit is named as the person responsible for assessment of progress in the National Maternity Hospital, just as she is also responsible for diagnosis of labour. The subjective element in interpretation is most pronounced when changes of staff occur; this possibility should be kept always in mind because it has a practical bearing on management, where a false impression of secondary arrest in progress is easily created.

Cervical dilatation

The degree of dilatation of cervix is recorded graphically on a partogram and plotted against hours after admission. Full dilatation is equated with 10 cm because this is the approximate diameter of a newborn baby's head. The time allotted is 10 hours. It follows that the slowest rate of dilatation acceptable is 1 cm each hour. The whole purpose of the partogram is to relate progress to passage of time in a visual manner which is readily intelligible, even to a lay person. Selected partograms are provided in Section II of this manual.

The extent to which rate of progress dominates all other aspects of labour should be noted. Partograms crammed with minute detail lose their visual impact; the result is that the main purpose of the exercise is defeated. Efforts to include every conceivable detail of every aspect of labour, whether relevant to the central issue or not, are counterproductive.

A clear pattern of dilatation should have emerged within 3 hours: on this basis it should be possible to predict the hour of delivery by simple linear projection in all but a few instances (see Figure 6.1). Close attention to progress during the early hours is the best insurance against difficulty later. The weight of emphasis currently placed on the first 3 hours of labour stands in sharp contrast with previous practice, when no worthwhile medical decision was considered necessary until a woman had been in labour for several hours, and complications had begun to threaten. Those belated decisions were concerned primarily with the rescue of mothers and babies from potentially dangerous predicaments that had developed over a protracted period in normal cases after admission to hospital. No serious thought was given to prevention.

Four hours is much too long to wait to discover that labour has not progressed since a previous examination, and it is much too long to wait to discover that treatment prescribed to accelerate slow progress after a previous examination has not been successful. Prolonged labour is far more likely to occur where pelvic examination is performed at infrequent and irregular intervals; infrequent and irregular pelvic examinations encourage a tolerant attitude to prolonged labour.

An unsatisfactory rate of dilatation of cervix during the early hours of labour is a clear expression of inefficient uterine action. The defect should be corrected without undue delay. This pattern of dilatation has no relevance whatever to cephalo-pelvic disproportion, a false association that has given rise to a great deal of confusion in the past. Treatment of inefficient uterine action is discussed in Chapter 8 and illustrated in Partograms 18 and 19 (see pp. 169 and 171, respectively).

Communication

One of the main benefits to accrue from pelvic assessment at relatively short intervals is the ability to keep the mother posted on the progress of events. Hopefully, it will have been explained to her beforehand, at antenatal classes, that the purpose of pelvic examination is to measure the speed at which the neck of her womb opens, because this effectively determines the length of her labour. In that case, she will already be familiar with the partogram. As time passes, the result of each examination is conveyed directly to her by the examiner as it is being entered on the partogram. As a lay person is not accustomed to think in terms of dilatation of cervix, but merely anxious to know when her baby will be born,

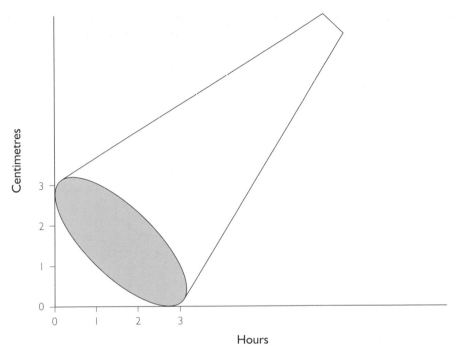

Figure 6.1.

attention is focused on the timescale. The need to be convinced that steady progress is being made, and to appreciate that there is a predictable end in sight, are matters of prime importance to the morale of all participants in the birth process.

The standard practice in the National Maternity Hospital is to inform every woman in labour of the projected time of her delivery as soon as a clear pattern of dilatation has emerged; this is information is usually imparted within 3 hours of admission. Time of delivery is stated to within 30 minutes. For example, at noon, the woman is told that her baby is expected at 4 o'clock in the afternoon, give or take a half hour. This information is updated after each pelvic examination. No pelvic examination is undertaken on a woman in labour without her direct involvement and in deference to her before, during and after the event. She must know the purpose of the examination and be the first to learn of the result. The onus rests squarely on the examiner to ensure that the woman genuinely understands the real meaning of what is being said. Platitudes, to the effect that 'all is well' or progress is 'as good as can be expected', are not tolerated. These inanities constitute an affront to the intelligence of women generally, and thus serve to undermine mutual confidence. Similarly, technical terms are strictly avoided. These are seen as a cloak for ignorance; an examiner who does not really comprehend the implications of the signs elicited is in no position to explain them to a third party and therefore retreats behind medical jargon.

Key Points

- Dilatation of cervix is the only measure of progress appropriate to the first stage of labour
- A clear pattern of dilatation should have emerged within 3 hours

Progress: Second Stage 7

The second stage of labour begins at full dilatation. In practice, this means when no part of the cervix is palpable at pelvic examination. For record purposes only, full dilatation is equated with 10 cm, because this is the approximate width of the mature fetal head. Progress in the second stage of labour is measured in terms of descent and rotation.

The contribution of the second stage to the total duration of labour is relatively small, because the second stage seldom lasts longer than 2 hours. The second stage of labour deserves particular attention because of the special risk of trauma. Although trauma is confined, virtually, to the second stage of labour, antecedent events are often highly relevant. With the notable exception of breech presentation, serious injury to the child is almost always associated with operative intervention to effect birth by traction, because the mother is unable, unwilling or, perhaps, not given the opportunity to deliver herself.

Such was the emphasis placed on full dilatation in previous times that it became generally accepted as the natural line of demarcation between abdominal and vaginal delivery. This is a serious fallacy, one fraught with gravest consequences. In practical terms, the second stage of labour is composed of two quite distinct phases: the first phase extends from full dilatation until the head reaches the pelvic floor, the second phase extends from then until the baby is born. These two phases are as different from each other as chalk is from cheese. The second stage of labour, in other words, is not a single entity.

Phase one

During phase one of the second stage of labour, the head is relatively high in the pelvis, the occiput may be in the transverse diameter, the vagina is not stretched and there is no inclination on the part of the mother to push. Neither the mother nor her attendants are aware of any significant change, and the fact that the cervix has reached full dilatation would pass entirely without notice unless, perchance, a vaginal examination was performed at this juncture. This phase is but a natural extension of the first stage of labour and care should not differ in any way. A woman with no inclination to push should not be urged to do so. If the woman has an urge to push in this phase rapid progress should be expected, otherwise active pushing should be discouraged. No attempt should be made to achieve vaginal delivery by traction; if the need for urgent delivery arises this should be by caesarean section. In terms of care, therefore, full dilatation of cervix is an event of academic interest only. This reservation applies to the time element also, a subject discussed in the following paragraph.

Phase two

Phase two of the second stage of labour begins when the head impacts on the floor of the pelvis, an event that coincides with a dramatic change in the demeanour of the mother. Vaginal delivery is virtually assured at this point, and whenever the need for intervention arises the ventouse, or standard obstetric forceps, can be used. The duration of this phase must be restricted because of the exceptional physical strain to which both mother and child are subjected by the compulsive urge to push. This is where the time factor becomes a vital consideration. There is no corresponding need to restrict the duration of phase one, because the element of exceptional physical strain does not apply.

Some of the most potentially dangerous misunderstandings in current obstetric practice stem from failure to draw a sharp distinction between these two phases of the second stage of labour. The classic example is when ventouse or forceps is applied as a matter of routine, simply because the cervix is known to be fully dilated for an arbitrary period. A difficult rotation is followed by strong traction to over-come soft tissue resistance. This leads to a diagnosis of cephalopelvic disproportion where none exists. The mother is exposed to the immediate risk of serious injury, and her future plans are prejudiced by prior committal to elective caesarean section on the basis of an incorrect interpretation of the sequence of events.

Key Points

- The second stage of labour is composed of two distinct phases
- Progress in the second stage of labour is assessed by descent, followed by rotation

Acceleration of Slow Labour   8

The most important decisions relating to management of labour are made during the first 3 hours. The decision to accelerate is one of these. Three hours after admission to a delivery unit, the course of labour should be set to the extent that it ought then to be possible to predict the approximate time of delivery in all but a few instances. The ability to predict the time of delivery at this comparatively early stage is of inestimable value to all who are involved in the birth process.

Procedure

Circumstances dictate that the decision to accelerate progress – like the diagnosis of labour – must be made by a midwife, because midwives, unlike obstetricians, are physically present in the delivery unit at all times. Crucial decisions on care in labour must not be allowed to go by default simply because women admit themselves in labour at inconvenient hours. The duty of the consultant obstetrician is to state clearly – preferably in writing – the basic rules of procedure and this should entail accepting responsibility for the outcome. Prolonged labour has been virtually eliminated from the National Maternity Hospital, mainly because the midwife in charge of the delivery unit knows precisely what to do, and when to do it. She knows, too, that no blame will attach to her in the event of an adverse outcome. This is a vital consideration, failing which no plan of action is likely to succeed. The procedure is outlined below.

First assessment

Progress is assessed, initially, at 2 hours after the diagnosis of labour (see *Partograms 4* and *11*, pp. 141 and 155, respectively). Artificial rupture of membranes is performed in all cases as soon as a firm diagnosis of labour is made. This procedure is carried out only in the delivery ward and if there is any doubt about the diagnosis of labour the decision to rupture the membranes is deferred for 1 hour. It is not a decision taken lightly.

    Apart from the fact that the nature of the liquor provides material evidence of the fetal condition and, therefore, should be ascertained in every case, there are four subsidiary reasons why the membranes are ruptured at this juncture:

- In the event of slow progress, rupture of membranes alone may be sufficient to accelerate (see *Partograms 17* and *21*, pp. 167 and 175, respectively).
- Oxytocin is not permitted if there is a suspicion of fetal distress, eg release of thick meconium at rupture of membranes.
- Oxytocin may be ineffective with intact membranes (see *Partogram 21*, p. 175).
- Theoretically, oxytocin may increase the risk of amniotic fluid infusion into the maternal circulation unless free drainage has been established.

Spontaneous rupture of membranes has already occurred in some 30% of women who admit themselves to this hospital in labour.

An oxytocin infusion is started unless significant progress – notionally 1 cm/hour – has been made. The decision to use oxytocin is taken by the midwife in charge, without reference to medical personnel (see *Partogram 18*, p. 169).

The following conditions must be fulfilled:

- The mother must be nulliparous.
- The presentation must be vertex.
- The fetus must be single.
- The membranes must be ruptured.
- There must be no evidence of fetal distress.

Special attention is drawn to the fact that oxytocin may not be given to a parous woman without authorization by a senior member of medical staff, who must then assume personal responsibility for the conduct of the case. The decision to give oxytocin to a parous woman cannot be taken by a midwife or junior doctor, nor can they be held responsible for the outcome.

Second assessment

Progress is assessed for the second time at 3 hours after admission (see *Partogram 4*, p. 141). A dramatic change is expected. It should now be possible to predict full dilatation, and consequent delivery, from a linear projection on the partogram (see *Partograms 4* and *18*, pp. 141 and 169, respectively).

Subsequent assessments

Further progress is assessed at intervals not exceeding 2 hours. In practice, the next examination is likely to be performed to confirm full dilatation, when the mother feels the urge to push (see *Partogram 18*, p. 169).

This makes a total of four pelvic examinations in the course of an average labour: at admission to confirm the diagnosis and to rupture the membranes, two further examinations in the early hours to assess progress and, finally, before the mother is allowed to push.

Slow progress

In the most unlikely event of failure to respond to oxytocin infusion, there are two possible explanations. First, the woman may not be in labour, because the initial diagnosis was wrong (see *Partogram 20*, p. 173). Second, the forewaters may be intact, despite the fact that liquor may have been seen to drain (see *Partogram 21*, p. 175). Once again, acceleration must not be confused with induction, where oxytocin frequently proves ineffective (see *Partograms 25* and *26*, pp. 183 and 185, respectively).

Slow progress in labour is almost always confined to women in whom the cervix is less than 2 cm dilated at admission. When the cervix is more than 2 cm dilated there are few problems: diagnosis is easy, progress is rapid, and spontaneous delivery is likely within a matter of hours. The extent to which the cervix is dilated at the time of admission is an accurate reflection of the quality of uterine action; contrary to popular belief, it bears little, if any, relationship to the number of hours a woman has spent in labour at home. Thirty percent of nulliparous women deliver themselves within 4 hours of admission in the National Maternity Hospital (see *Table 8*, p. 209).

Secondary arrest

In the much less likely event of secondary arrest in progress during the first stage of labour, when dilatation has been satisfactory in the early hours but comes to a virtual standstill later, the same procedure is followed. Oxytocin is infused in a similar manner. Caesarean section is undertaken after a limited period of time unless normal progress has resumed. This unusual pattern of dilatation raises the question of cephalopelvic disproportion for the first time and the diagnosis is taken as confirmed should the pattern persist after uterine action has been restored.

Secondary arrest in progress may not occur until the second stage of labour when, after full dilatation has been achieved, the head does not descend. Failure of descent is the clinical manifestation of 'dystocia' during the second stage of labour and should be seen as the counterpart of failure to dilate during the first stage.

Operative delivery

The conventional method of treatment of slow progress in the second stage of labour is operative delivery. Ventouse or forceps is applied in three distinct clinical circumstances which are quite different from one another, as follows.

First, the instruments may be applied as soon as full dilatation is achieved after a long first stage of labour. The declared purpose is to bring the mother's ordeal to a speedy conclusion, or to anticipate fetal distress based sometimes on slender evidence. This being phase one of the second stage, the head is still high in the transverse diameter of the pelvis. Delivery entails rotation, frequently with rotational forceps, followed by strong traction to overcome soft tissue resistance, because although the cervix is sufficiently dilated, the vagina is most certainly not. This manoeuvre is, arguably, the main source of serious injury to both mother and child in contemporary obstetrics. Perpetuation of the manoeuvre is based on the archaic proposition that full dilatation of cervix is the natural line of demarcation between abdominal and vaginal delivery. This situation must change. It must be recognized that a case of this nature would fare much better if full dilatation was never achieved. At least this would protect against misguided attempts at forcible vaginal delivery. Forceps, or ventouse, are not used during the first stage of labour.

Second, the instruments may be applied when uterine action fails, as a secondary phenomenon, after a normal first stage. The head remains high, in the transverse position, because the driving force is inadequate. From the standpoint of vaginal delivery, the prospect is the same as in the previous paragraph: the woman remains stranded in phase one of the second stage of labour.

Third, the instruments may be applied after the head has reached the floor of the pelvis when, despite good uterine action, the mother is unable to overcome the formidable obstacle presented by the levator muscles through her own efforts. Not infrequently, this impasse arises because the mother is emotionally and physically exhausted after a long first stage, or mentally confused by a large dosage of drugs. She has, however, made the critical transition from phase one to phase two of the second stage of labour, to the point at which delivery with ventouse or forceps is a comparatively safe procedure. The vagina, as well as the cervix, is now dilated.

Oxytocin as alternative

Conventional methods of care in phase one of the second stage of labour offer a straight choice between caesarean section and difficult vaginal operative delivery. Faced with these alternatives, preference should be for caesarean section, in the interest of all parties concerned.

There is, however, a third option available: oxytocin. The relatively common clinical problem described above provides one of the most impressive examples of the constructive use of oxytocin across the whole of obstetrics. An oxytocin infusion begun in the second stage of labour restores normal uterine action; this causes the head to descend to the pelvic floor and also, hopefully, to rotate at that level. The result is that a difficult vaginal operative delivery is transformed into an easy assisted delivery, if not, indeed, a spontaneous delivery. There is no better practical illustration of one of the basic concepts of Active Management of Labour: that delivery by propulsion is preferable to delivery by traction. The intelligent use of oxytocin introduced in the second stage of labour has made an important contribution to reduction in the incidence of trauma to both mothers and infants in this hospital in recent years (see *Partogram 19* and *Table 5*, pp. 171 and 203, respectively).

Key Points

- Duration of labour is determined by rate of dilatation of cervix in the early hours
- Dilatation must be monitored during the first 3 hours by regular pelvic examinations
- Early acceleration with oxytocin ensures efficient uterine action and normal progress in nulliparous women
- Oxytocin should be considered as a possible alternative to operative delivery in the second stage of labour
- Oxytocin should not be given to a parous woman without authorization at the highest level

Oxytocin in Labour   9

Oxytocin is one of the most specific therapeutic agents available in medicine. Properly used, it can also be one of the safest. The therapeutic effect of oxytocin is to cause the cervix to dilate during the first stage, and the head to descend during the second stage. This sequential action is almost invariably achieved. Indeed, the effect of oxytocin is so predictable that whenever the cervix does not dilate during the first stage, by far the most likely explanation is that the woman is not in labour. Failure of the cervix to dilate in response to oxytocin constitutes a clear indication to review the diagnosis of labour, and here again it is necessary to emphasize the fundamental difference between induction of labour and acceleration of labour, because oxytocin is not nearly so predictable in initiating the process as it is in accelerating progress after labour has already started. The only other situations where the cervix may sometimes fail to dilate is where there has been an inordinate delay before commencement of oxytocin or the membranes remain intact.

Explicit rules

The rules that govern the use of oxytocin are quite explicit; furthermore, they are rigidly enforced. Extensive practical experience has shown that these rules provide a highly effective series of safeguards:

- A standard concentration of 10 units of oxytocin in 1 litre of normal saline is used in all circumstances.
- The total dose of oxytocin received may not exceed 10 units.
- The rate of infusion may not exceed 60 drops per minute.*
- Infusion of 1 litre at the prescribed rate imposes a time limit of 6 hours.

The only variable factor is the rate of infusion; this begins at 10 drops and increases by 10 drops, at intervals of 15 minutes, to a maximum of 60 drops. The rate of infusion attains the maximum of 60 drops in the shortest time – 75 minutes – in almost every instance. Evidence of fetal distress is the only absolute bar to this step-by-step method of progression.

---

* The drip set used conforms with the British standard specification, which requires that 15–20 drops are equivalent to 1 ml. The maximum dose of oxytocin at 60 drops, therefore, is 40 milliunits/minute.

Oxytocin infused in this manner is so uniformly successful in accelerating progress in labour that it can be used too often; for this reason it should be kept under constant review and audited as with all other obstetric procedures.

Hypertonic uterine action

The personal nurse – who accompanies everyone in labour – records each contraction as it occurs after oxytocin has started. The partogram is used for this purpose: the timescale is divided into intervals of 15 minutes; the optimum number of contractions in this period is five. To guard against hypertonus the number of contractions is not permitted to exceed seven in 15 minutes under any circumstance.

Special care is taken to ensure that the mother does not control the drip. In practice, this occurs when the attendant reduces the rate of infusion simply because the mother complains of pain, which is, of course, to be expected. Such indecision is a common manifestation of a low level of confidence in the system, which usually derives from imprecise instructions or lack of trust.

Special equipment

An infusion pump may be used as an alternative to a simple gravity feed, but automation of this nature should not become a mechanical substitute for personal attention. Moreover, it is a mistake to think that a precise dose of oxytocin, in milliunits per minute, offers any material advantage. This is an item of utmost practical importance in centres where special equipment may not be available.

The overall contribution of a personal nurse to a woman in labour extends far beyond supervision of oxytocin, while the response to the suggestion that it is not feasible to provide personal attention on such a scale is to remind the reader that this recommendation emanates from an exceptionally busy unit.

Causes of confusion

The situation with regard to oxytocin in some centres is difficult to comprehend. There are several consultant obstetricians, each with a fixed preference for a different regimen for which there is no factual basis. Intuitively, it seems, one consultant feels that 2.5 units of oxytocin is best, another 5 units and another 10 units, and to confuse the matter still further, some use all three consecutively in the same case. This bizarre example of therapeutics, where the dose of a drug is altered both in terms of concentration and in rate of administration, can have few counterparts in medicine. Is it any wonder that those called upon to supervise similar cases in adjoining beds, who are prescribed different concentrations of the same drug to treat the same disorder, should feel utterly confused? And when these complexities are compounded by ominous references to possible cephalopelvic disproportion, rupture of uterus and injury to the child, their position becomes virtually untenable. The only sensible course open to a responsible person placed in such an intolerable position would be to reduce the rate of infusion to an ineffectual level, which is not sufficient to dilate the cervix, and to record hypertonic uterine action or fetal distress as the reason for doing so. This is what frequently occurs in practice, thus giving rise to the mistaken impression that oxytocin is sometimes not an effective method of resolving the problem of slow labour. Staff in the National Maternity Hospital are indemnified against cephalopelvic disproportion, rupture of uterus and injury to the child. Care is taken to avoid reference to these subjects altogether in the present context. Criticism is reserved for those who fail to act decisively to restrict the duration of labour.

Water intoxication

The only direct toxic effect of oxytocin is water intoxication. This classical syndrome – which may result in convulsions, coma and even death – is due to an intrinsic antidiuretic effect of oxytocin, which results in reabsorption of salt-free water from renal tubules. As the name implies, water intoxication is related directly to volume of fluid available. The possibility arises when more than 3 litres of salt-free fluid are administered by the intravenous route. This simply cannot occur when the rules, as previously stated, are followed; the fact that the volume of fluid is restricted to 1 litre provides an absolute guarantee against water intoxication. Naturally, careful notice must also be taken of alternative sources of fluid given intravenously, as for example by an anaesthetist in conjunction with epidural anaesthesia. This can be an important source of additional fluid, especially when epidural anaesthesia is misused as a cover for prolonged labour; the longer the labour the greater the volume of fluid infused. Oral fluids do not contribute to the problem of water intoxication because these are regulated by the mother, not imposed upon her.

Water intoxication is far more likely to occur when oxytocin is used to induce labour, because all too often induction is allowed to continue for an indefinite period, during which an excessive volume of salt-free fluid may be infused unnoticed.

Neonatal jaundice

An association between oxytocin and neonatal jaundice has attracted some attention. Studies in the National Maternity Hospital have confirmed that there is an increase in the incidence of neonatal jaundice in cases treated with oxytocin, but they have also shown that this increase is confined to cases in which oxytocin is used to induce labour. There is no increase in cases in which oxytocin is used to accelerate labour already started. The overall increase in the incidence of neonatal jaundice associated with oxytocin, therefore, is a reflection of relative prematurity which results from interruption of the course of pregnancy before its natural conclusion; it is not a direct toxic effect of oxytocin. This constitutes yet another example of the need to draw a sharp distinction between induction and acceleration of labour.[5]

Trauma

For many years it has been taught that oxytocin increases the risk of trauma to both mother and child, especially where there may be an element of cephalopelvic disproportion. There is no foundation for this proposition in nulliparous women. In nulliparous women the opposite is true because efficient uterine action reduces the need for traction, which is the real cause of trauma. There was no case of rupture of the uterus in more than 100 000 consecutive nulliparous women delivered in this hospital during the 40 years under review. There were five cases of traumatic intracranial haemorrhage in cephalic presentations not delivered by forceps. The incidence of traumatic intracranial haemorrhage in cephalic presentations showed a sharp decline after the present policy of prevention of prolonged labour was introduced. The fundamental difference between nulliparous and parous women must be emphasized once again, since oxytocin is a potent cause of rupture of uterus in parous women. The subject of trauma is considered at greater length in Chapter 14 (see also *Tables 4* and *5*, pp. 201 and 203, respectively).

Hypoxia

Hypoxia is an entirely different proposition. Every contraction of the uterus reduces circulation through the placenta, even during the course of normal labour. This presents no serious challenge to a fetus who starts labour with a normal placenta, but it can have grave consequences where placental function is already impaired. A fetus with normal placental function is well equipped to withstand the stress of normal labour, unless an accident like prolapse of cord should occur. The fetus who is likely to suffer from hypoxia during the course of normal labour is the fetus whose placental function was impaired before labour began, hence the importance of ascertaining the nature of the liquor at an early stage. To the fetus, the consequences are the same whether the natural action of the uterus is sufficient to dilate the cervix, or inefficient uterine action is corrected with oxytocin. Since the purpose of oxytocin is to simulate normal uterine action, it follows that circulation through the placenta is reduced; in this sense it is inevitable that oxytocin should contribute to the problem of hypoxia. However, hypoxia is not a direct toxic effect of oxytocin; it is a by-product of efficient uterine action.

Key Points

- Oxytocin is effective in the treatment of inefficient uterine action; it can almost uniformly be safely used in nulliparous women

- Oxytocin should not be used if there is evidence of fetal hypoxia

- Oxytocin should only be used with utmost caution in parous women

- The incidence of oxytocin should be kept under critical review

Normal and Abnormal Labour (Dystocia) 10

It may seem strange that the basic parameters of normal labour, to which all who are concerned with obstetric care should consciously aspire, are seldom, if ever, clearly defined. Although it would be difficult to gain universal acceptance on every minute detail, an attempt to achieve this would be an immensely rewarding exercise. An agreed definition of normal labour should be posted in a prominent position in every delivery unit – and classroom – to serve as a clear statement of common purpose. The subject should be considered in broad outline, with controversial issues best avoided.

In the National Maternity Hospital labour is classified as normal when a baby is born vaginally, by the efforts of the mother, within a reasonable timespan, provided no harm befalls either party as a result of their experience. Twelve hours is regarded as a reasonable timespan.

Conversely, labour is classified as abnormal when delivery is by caesarean section, or vaginally by the efforts of the doctor, when duration exceeds 12 hours, or when some harmful effect befalls either mother or child. Induction of labour is designated abnormal, as are all operative deliveries. This is not to say that induction, caesarean section and low forceps, or ventouse, are not practised, but rather practised with discretion, and always as the lesser of two evils. Rotational forceps, however, are not used.

Although at first sight these definitions may appear somewhat unrealistic to those accustomed to think of childbirth in terms of technical procedures, developments in the National Maternity Hospital over 40 years have shown that this viewpoint is perfectly tenable.

Abnormal labour, or dystocia, has three possible causes: inefficient uterine action, occipitoposterior position and cephalopelvic disproportion (see *Figure 10.1*). These correspond with faults in the passage, in the passenger and in the forces. Significantly, the order of priority is reversed. Attention is again directed to the fact that the term 'cephalopelvic disproportion', as used throughout this manual, refers only to nulliparous women and that malpresentations, malformations and twins are covered specifically in Chapter 3. These complications may give rise to obstructed labour, which constitutes an entirely different clinical syndrome from cephalopelvic disproportion.

There is bound to be a subjective element involved in the differential diagnosis between the three possible causes of abnormal labour in individual cases. Occipitoposterior position is the clear exception because, in a negative sense at least, it can be excluded at pelvic examination. The main problem therefore lies between inefficient uterine action and cephalopelvic disproportion. In practice, the differential diagnosis between these two causes of abnormal labour continues to be based largely on personal preference. Local custom frequently determines which cases of abnormal labour, or dystocia, are attributed to cephalopelvic disproportion, while X-ray pelvimetries are used to bolster opinions which are largely preconceived. This dubious method of procedure is still very evident in the wide variation in the reported incidence of cephalopelvic disproportion in maternity units which are located in the same geographical region and which appear similar in all other respects. The reported incidence of cephalopelvic disproportion is merely a statement of the number of caesarean sections included under that heading on an arbitrary basis. This is an implausible method of estimating the true prevalence of a disease, and obviously one on which no reliance can be placed.

Traditionally, cephalopelvic disproportion has been taught to medical students and pupil midwives as the most important feature of abnormal labour. This seemingly arose out of genuine concern that serious harm might befall both mother and child should the condition be overlooked. As previously stated, this is a fundamental mistake, one for which there is absolutely no clinical support. There can be little doubt that the error arose because cephalopelvic disproportion in nulliparous women, and obstructed labour in parous women, were not recognized as distinct entities, with different causes, different treatment and different results. Even more important in this context was failure to recognize that the nulliparous uterus is virtually immune to rupture, whereas the parous uterus is rupture prone.

Probably the most significant outcome of Active Management of Labour is that effective uterine action is sought in every case, with the result that the problem of cephalopelvic disproportion has been isolated for the first time. Now the differential diagnosis between inefficient uterine action, cephalopelvic disproportion and occipitoposterior position can be made by a simple process of exclusion. Given a cervix which dilates progressively, and an occiput which is not posterior, a diagnosis of cephalopelvic disproportion can confidently be made.

The causes of abnormal labour, or dystocia, are discussed in Chapters 11, 12 and 13; these should be read in conjunction with this chapter.

Key Points

- A clear working definition of normal labour should be posted in a prominent position in every delivery unit, to serve as a statement of common purpose

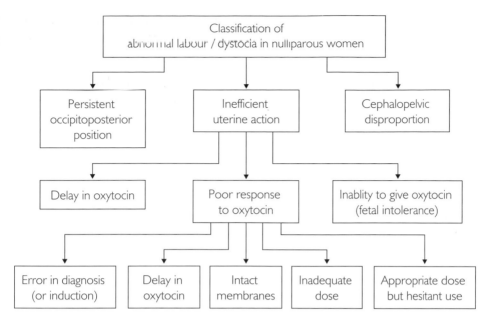

Figure 10.1 Classification of abnormal labour (dystocia) in nulliparous women.

Inefficient Uterine Action   11

Inefficient uterine action is far and away the most common complication of labour in nulliparous women. This is certainly not so in parous women. A diagnosis of inefficient uterine action in a parous woman should always be viewed with the gravest suspicion, because the parous uterus is a highly efficient organ with much less resistance to overcome. Slow progress in a parous woman may well be an expression of obstruction, and obstructed labour in a parous woman is much the commonest cause of rupture of uterus. That there are essential differences between nulliparous and parous labour needs constant reiteration. The present chapter, on inefficient uterine action, refers to nulliparous women only; the contents should be applied to parous women with extreme caution.

Definitions

The sole function of the uterus during the first stage of labour is to cause the cervix to dilate. During the second stage of labour, the sole function of the uterus is to cause the head to descend to the level of the pelvic floor. These disparate functions must not be confused. Pressure on the pelvic floor activates the reflex action of voluntary muscles, which in turn cause the baby to be born. The efficiency of the uterus during labour can be gauged only by its ability to complete these specific functions, each within a reasonable timescale. In other words, the efficiency of the uterus can be measured only in terms of results achieved. These results correlate equally poorly with the subjective element of pain as felt by the mother, and with the objective strength of contractions as assessed by her attendant. The success or failure of treatment of inefficient uterine action must not be evaluated in this manner.

Acceptance of oxytocin

Although the means, in the form of oxytocin, have long been available, a systematic approach to the problem of inefficient uterine action has been slow to emerge. The reasons for this delay seem to have been as follows:

- As the first step towards solution of a problem is accurate definition, failure to submit the syndrome of abnormal labour, or dystocia, to detailed analysis rendered a solution virtually impossible.

59

- Inefficient uterine action, which is by far the most common cause of abnormal labour, was itself complicated by being subdivided into two distinct types: hypotonic and hypertonic inertia. This subdivision was coupled with the warning that although stimulation with oxytocin could be beneficial to the former, it could be detrimental to the latter. There is no basis for this assertion: in clinical practice inefficient uterine action is a single entity and is uniformly responsive to stimulation with oxytocin.
- Improving inefficient uterine action was further inhibited by the proposition, which amounted almost to an article of faith, that stimulation of the uterus in circumstances in which there was even the faintest possibility of cephalopelvic disproportion could result in serious injury to both mother and child. As cephalopelvic disproportion can never, strictly speaking, be excluded wholly until labour has come to a successful conclusion, this caveat ensured that oxytocin could not be used to proper effect for fear of dire consequences. Because labour could not be brought to a successful conclusion without efficient uterine action, this gave rise to a classic example of a chicken and egg situation. The result was therapeutic paralysis.

Clinical types

Typically, inefficient uterine action presents as slow dilatation of cervix which continues from the very onset of labour. This persistent pattern of slow dilatation should lead to early diagnosis and prompt treatment, long before dehydration, ketosis or other evidence of physical and mental exhaustion can make an appearance. Moreover, the cervix of a woman in labour is so predictably responsive to stimulation with oxytocin that, whenever the rate of dilatation does not accelerate sharply, the initial diagnosis of labour is almost certainly wrong. Where little attention is paid to diagnosis of labour such cases are commonplace; they may even create an impression that oxytocin is not a reliable method of treatment. Alternatively, this false impression may derive from the popular confusion between acceleration and induction, where there is no clear indication as to when labour begins. It is of the utmost importance to appreciate that slow dilatation of cervix, as a primary phenomenon, is not at all suggestive of cephalopelvic disproportion.

Much less frequently, inefficient uterine action may develop as a secondary phenomenon, in which case it presents as arrest in dilatation of cervix late in the first stage of labour, after there has been a normal beginning. Secondary arrest in dilatation of cervix is indeed suggestive of cephalopelvic disproportion but, because inefficient uterine action is still a more likely cause, individuals should be given oxytocin for a limited period before resort is made to caesarean section.

Finally, inefficient uterine action may not develop until the second stage of labour, in which case it presents as failure of the head to descend after full dilatation has been achieved. The clinical situation is identical with that discussed in the previous paragraph; hence, oxytocin should be given for a limited period before resort is made to caesarean section. Forcible vaginal delivery with ventouse or forceps should certainly not be undertaken at this juncture, simply because the cervix has reached full dilatation (see *Partograms 12, 13, 14, 15* and *16*, pp. 157, 159, 161, 163 and 165, respectively).

Key Points

- Efficient uterine action is the key to normal labour

- Efficient uterine action can safely be assured through judicious use of oxytocin, with one overriding qualification: that a clear distinction be maintained between nulliparous and parous women

- Ensuring efficient uterine action in every nulliparous woman isolates the problem of cephalopelvic disproportion

Cephalopelvic Disproportion 12

The concept of cephalopelvic disproportion has coloured attitudes to childbirth for a very long time.[6] The main reason for this is that cephalopelvic disproportion is coupled, in the collective subconscious of obstetricians, with the threat of rupture of the uterus and injury to the child. Hence it may come as a surprise to learn that in the whole of recorded clinical experience there is no factual basis for either contention. Of course, this is to presume that the term 'cephalopelvic disproportion' is used correctly to refer to nulliparous women only, and not extended, incorrectly, to include parous women. Rupture of uterus is a calamity that befalls parous women with obstructed labour, usually caused by malpresentations; it does not affect nulliparous women with cephalopelvic disproportion. Moreover, injury to a firstborn child is associated almost exclusively with instrumental delivery. The subject of trauma is discussed at greater length in Chapter 14.

There may have been good reason for the widespread concern about cephalopelvic disproportion when rickets was a common disease, but this situation no longer exists. In retrospect, it now seems to have been an unfortunate coincidence that when X-ray pelvimetry was perfected in the 1950s, the social conditions that gave rise to rickets were eradicated. This has served to perpetuate a preoccupation with a condition which is hardly ever seen nowadays. At that time, X-ray pelvimetry seemed to provide an objective scientific basis for the study of cephalopelvic disproportion because it reduced the issue to a simple question of shape and size, features which could be accurately portrayed. A diagnosis of contracted pelvis and, by inference, cephalopelvic disproportion, was compared with that of an orthopaedic fracture: a straightforward combination of modern equipment and technical expertise. It seemed all too reasonable to assume that accurate measurements of her pelvis could only be helpful to a woman facing childbirth for the first time, just as it would have seemed perverse to suggest that such measurements could, in the event, become a liability. But this has proved in practice to be the case.

The standard procedure in those days was to combine digital assessment of pelvis with a head-fitting test in the case of every nulliparous woman in whom the head had not engaged at, say, 38 weeks. This was combined with X-ray pelvimetry. A formal decision was then made between delivery by elective caesarean section and 'trial of labour'. Frequently this crucial decision, which could have permanent repercussions on a woman's lifestyle, was made, albeit indirectly, by a radiologist who had never even seen the patient. The entire birth process was dominated by architectural nuances.

A trial of labour was carefully documented in advance. Antenatal notes included predictions that were frequently pessimistic and always cautionary in tone. Nowhere was it appreciated that a trial of labour might fail simply because the outcome was prejudiced beforehand, or because an intolerable burden of responsibility was placed on midwives and junior doctors by these reservations so freely expressed by their senior colleagues. There was an absolute bar on the use of oxytocin, because it was taken for granted that stimulation of the uterus in the presence of suspected cephalopelvic disproportion could easily result in serious damage to mother or child. Moreover, whenever the uterus did not function effectively to dilate the cervix, this was seen as a protective mechanism which served only to confirm the original suspicion. Finally, a diagnosis of cephalopelvic disproportion once made was permanent in its effect, so that later children were delivered by elective caesarean section without further consideration. This method of procedure had important long-term implications for the woman and her family, which attracted surprisingly little attention.

On an historical note, it was in the National Maternity Hospital that the operation of symphisiotomy was revived in the 1940s, to offset the commitment to repeat caesarean sections in young mothers with a diagnosis of cephalopelvic disproportion. This practice continued for more than 20 years until Active Management of Labour was introduced in the 1960s. This development ensured efficient uterine action for every nulliparous woman in labour. Soon it became apparent that most women previously treated by symphisiotomy, or caesarean section, after failed trial of labour suffered not from cephalopelvic disproportion, but from inefficient uterine action. Within a few years the recorded incidence of cephalopelvic disproportion had fallen to a small fraction of the previous level. Meanwhile, however, the operation had been transported to other centres, mainly in Africa, where it is still practised.

Definition

Cephalopelvic disproportion is a term used only in the context of first-time mothers with normal, vertex presentations. This restricted use of the term is considered a matter of fundamental importance to the elucidation of the problem. The term cephalopelvic disproportion is, advisedly, not used in the context of later births, nor does it include malpresentations, or certain malformations, whatever the mother's parity. The term 'obstructed labour' is used to describe a completely different clinical entity which directly involves the fetus, such as brow or shoulder presentation or hydrocephalus. Here the capacity of the pelvis is not the central issue. Obstructed labour, in a parous woman, is a much more dangerous proposition than cephalopelvic disproportion in a nulliparous woman, because it is all too likely to lead to serious trauma. Rupture of uterus becomes almost inevitable should the obstruction escape notice and oxytocin be infused to stimulate the parous uterus which is efficient by nature. The mistaken belief that a similar fate might befall a nulliparous woman with cephalopelvic disproportion, or indeed obstruction, stems from the general failure to draw a clear distinction between mothers on grounds of parity.

Diagnosis

No consideration whatever is given to the possibility of cephalopelvic disproportion in the course of routine antenatal care in the National Maternity Hospital. All reference to the subject is consciously excluded. No mention is made in case notes, in the firm belief that this can only have an adverse influence on the eventual outcome. The pelvis is not assessed by clinical means, nor is X-ray pelvimetry practised. The result is that elective caesarean section is almost never performed for this indication and, in particular, the term 'trial of labour' is studiously avoided at all times.

The possibility of cephalopelvic disproportion is raised for the first time after the course of labour has proved abnormal. Abnormal labour unfolds as the cervix fails to dilate progressively during the first stage, or the head fails to descend during the second stage. Slow progress early in labour (i.e. as a primary event) is interpreted invariably as an expression of inefficient uterine action, whereas slow progress as a secondary event (i.e. late in labour) is interpreted sometimes as an expression of cephalopelvic disproportion. Nonetheless, a diagnosis of cephalopelvic disproportion is not seriously entertained until oxytocin has been infused for a limited period in order to exclude inefficient uterine action which remains the more likely cause even of secondary arrest. A presumptive diagnosis of cephalopelvic disproportion is made when progress remains unsatisfactory under these conditions, provided that the occiput is not posterior. These are the clinical circumstances in which caesarean section for cephalopelvic disproportion is undertaken. No attempt is made to anticipate these events, because attempts to anticipate a diagnosis of cephalopelvic disproportion led to unnecessary surgical intervention in previous years (see *Partogram 23*, p. 179).

Even so, the final conclusion is postponed until the puerperium when, for the purpose of audit, every case of dystocia is formally reviewed. A differential diagnosis between inefficient uterine action, cephalopelvic disproportion and occipitoposterior position is made in the light of all the evidence available.

Also for the purpose of medical records, a diagnosis of cephalopelvic disproportion is positively excluded in each case in which labour is classified as normal, because vaginal delivery has been achieved within 12 hours and there has been no significant injury to mother or child. This means that a formal decision, either for or against a diagnosis of cephalopelvic disproportion, is made for every nulliparous woman delivered. The incidence of cephalopelvic disproportion, based on this comprehensive method of selection, has remained stable at 1 in 250 nulliparous women, approximately, for many years. Yet despite this exceptionally low figure, one in every two cases in which a diagnosis of cephalopelvic disproportion was made had a subsequent vaginal delivery in this hospital. Cephalopelvic disproportion, therefore, is clearly not a common disorder where rigorous standards of diagnosis are applied.

Pelvic deformity

Pelvic deformity is considered to be a separate disorder, with less than 1 in 1000 women being affected. Almost invariably, the deformity is caused either by a limp in childhood or by a crush injury in adult life. Diagnosis presents no problem as individuals declare themselves, either by their gait or by their history of a road traffic accident. These are virtually the only cases delivered by elective caesarean section for reasons of pelvic architecture.

Change in practice

Over recent decades no single aspect of obstetric practice in the National Maternity Hospital has undergone such radical change as the attitude towards cephalopelvic disproportion. The change has come about as a result of a combination of factors, chief amongst which are: insistence on the precise use of terms, realization that efficient uterine action is the key to normal birth, and conclusive evidence that oxytocin can be used safely in nulliparous women. It has become abundantly clear that all efforts to anticipate a diagnosis of cephalopelvic disproportion are not only misguided, they result in a rate of intervention grossly in excess of the true prevalence of the condition. This represents a classic example of a clinical situation where application of the generally laudable principle of prevention becomes counterproductive in its effects. Hence the term 'trial of labour' has been deleted from our vocabulary, and antenatal pelvimetry is no longer practised. Not even short stature is regarded any longer with suspicion, since small mothers generally give birth to small babies. This observation seems to have global application, as, for example, in Asia and Africa where western observers tend to place undue emphasis on short stature, without directing equal attention to low birth weight.

Key Points

- The term cephalopelvic disproportion applies to nulliparous women

- A prospective diagnosis of cephalopelvic disproportion is not entertained

- A diagnosis of cephalopelvic disproportion is only considered after efficient uterine action has been assured for a limited period

- No single aspect of obstetric practice has undergone such radical change as the attitude towards cephalopelvic disproportion

Occipitoposterior Position   13

Persistent occipitoposterior position is the third and only other possible cause of abnormal labour, or dystocia. The clinical problems posed are very similar to those associated with cephalopelvic disproportion. However, there is one important difference: it is possible to determine the position of the occiput by pelvic examination and it can be confirmed at caesarean section. Diagnosis, in this limited sense, is a straightforward procedure.[7]

Care in labour

The same pragmatic approach is adopted to occipitoposterior position as to cephalopelvic disproportion. No attention is paid to position of occiput during the final weeks of pregnancy and, to avoid giving rise to the impression that position may have an adverse effect on the course of labour, no record is kept at antenatal clinics. As with cephalopelvic disproportion, experience has shown that the greater the emphasis on the possibility, the more likely it is that difficulties will follow. The anxious doctor creates problems in both cases.

The clinical significance of posterior position does not come into question until the course of labour has already proved abnormal. This becomes evident when the cervix ceases to dilate during the first stage, or the head fails to descend during the second stage. Slow progress as a primary event, early in labour, is always interpreted as an expression of inefficient uterine action, whereas slow progress as a secondary event, i.e. late in labour, is sometimes interpreted as an expression of cephalopelvic disproportion and sometimes of occipitoposterior position. Even at this late juncture inefficient uterine action is still the most likely cause. Secondary arrest of progress that does not respond to oxytocin, given for a limited period, is attributed to malposition when the occiput is posterior and to cephalopelvic disproportion otherwise. Caesarean section is performed in either event, unless the cervix is fully dilated. Rotational forceps has no place in modern obstetric practice.

In clinical practice, the most dangerous aspect of persistent posterior position emerges during the second stage of labour, when the temptation to opt for vaginal delivery seems almost irresistible. Equating full dilatation with the point of no return in labour, when operative vaginal delivery becomes a challenge to manual dexterity, may lead to forcible rotation and extraction, the manoeuvre which, arguably, carries the greatest risk of trauma to both mother and child in contemporary obstetrics. A case of occipitoposterior position that persists for more than a limited period of time, having excluded inefficient uterine action, into the second stage of labour is delivered by caesarean section without regard to the fact that the cervix is fully dilated, unless the head is on the pelvic floor and manual rotation can be performed easily, or vaginal delivery be effected face to pubis. Forceps are not used to rotate, nor is the head ever displaced upwards for this purpose.

Transverse arrest

The term 'transverse arrest' is widely misconstrued. The normal position of the occiput is in the transverse diameter of the pelvis until the head reaches the level of the ischial spines, which mark the junction between the midstrait and the outlet of the bony structure. The ischial spines also mark the level of transition between phase one and phase two of the second stage of labour, described in Chapter 7, because they provide the attachments of the levator ani muscles which form the floor of the birth canal. At this level the reflex action of voluntary muscles is activated and forward rotation of occiput normally occurs. Rotation is effected by the combined action of uterine and voluntary muscles; when it fails to occur it is because this composite force is not equal to the task. Hence, arrest in the transverse diameter of the pelvis is not, as the term may seem to imply, the result of physical obstruction but rather the expression of inadequate driving force. Transverse arrest is not the cause of delay: it is the result.

The appropriate action in the case of transverse arrest, therefore, is that for delay in second stage. In the case of midtransverse arrest, so-called because the head remains above the level of the ischial spines, oxytocin is given to improve the action of the uterus and thus propel the head downwards to the level at which rotation naturally occurs. In the case of deep transverse arrest, so-called because the head is already at the level of the ischial spines, manual rotation and a simple vaginal operative delivery is permissible. No attempt is made to rotate, and subsequently extract, a head arrested in the midstrait of the pelvis; caesarean section is performed whenever the need for delivery arises in such circumstances.

The widespread misunderstanding that exists in respect of the significance of transverse arrest is reflected in the exaggerated attention paid to minor variations in shape and size of pelvis in centres where antenatal pelvimetry is still common practice. There is an unwarranted assumption that prominent ischial spines may cause deep transverse arrest, with the result that forecasts are made of likely trouble at the pelvic outlet long before labour begins. This is a characteristic feature of the mechanical approach to childbirth, where shape and size of pelvis, rather than functional efficiency of uterus, are the main focus of attention.

Results

Position of occiput is recorded as having an adverse effect on outcome in 1 in every 250 nulliparous women delivered in this hospital. By mere coincidence, this is the same figure quoted for cephalopelvic disproportion in Chapter 12. In effect, this means that approximately 8 in every 1000 nulliparous women – less than 1% – do not achieve safe vaginal delivery within a reasonable period of time as a consequence of one or other condition. The differential diagnosis is based almost entirely on the position of occiput at the point of delivery and is made, therefore, in retrospect. Although, inevitably, there is some degree of overlap between the two conditions, this does not affect the care advised in labour.

Key Points

- There is a close similarity between persistent occipitoposterior position and cephalopelvic disproportion in clinical practice

- Neither condition should be diagnosed before efficient uterine action has been assured for a limited time

- The term 'transverse arrest' should be discarded; it is a misnomer based on a misunderstanding of the natural process of descent and rotation during the course of normal labour

Trauma 14

Trauma in labour should be considered as a single entity, because the circumstances that give rise to trauma in the mother are usually the same as those that give rise to trauma in the child. These arise late in labour and are almost invariably associated with operative intervention at the point of delivery. Breech presentation is an exception: trauma in breech presentation is confined to the fetus and is inherent in the mode of delivery.

Injury to mother

Rupture of uterus is the classic example of serious trauma to the mother. This catastrophe is not likely to escape notice because it may result in blood transfusion and hysterectomy. The first reported case in the medical literature of rupture of uterus in a nulliparous woman, which was not associated with manipulation, occurred in a woman who was treated with oxytocin under cover of epidural anaesthesia, in the course of a labour that was allowed to continue for more than 50 hours.[8] The interest in this particular case is that it was reported for the express purpose of refuting our statement that the nulliparous uterus is virtually immune to rupture, except by manipulation. It could have been presented much more suitably as a bizarre exception to prove that general rule. There was, in fact, no case of ruptured uterus in more than 100 000 consecutive nulliparous women delivered in the National Maternity Hospital during the period under review, despite extensive use of oxytocin to accelerate progress in some 35 000 nulliparous women, in both first and second stages of labour (see *Table 4*, p. 201).

Laceration of cervix, rupture of vault, spiral tears of vagina and injury to anal sphincter and rectum are somewhat less dramatic manifestations of serious trauma to the mother which also may entail significant haemorrhage, blood transfusion and extensive surgical repair. Although not so easy to quantify accurately in numerical terms, these injuries are likewise associated almost exclusively with vaginal operative delivery, especially where forceps are used for the purpose of rotation in phase one of the second stage of labour.

Examples of surgical trauma to the mother include episiotomy and caesarean section. Caesarean sections performed at full dilatation in order to avoid difficult vaginal operative deliveries may themselves result in significant haemorrhage, blood transfusion and surgical repair.

Injury to child

Rupture of tentorium cerebelli is the classic example of serious trauma to the child. This lesion, which results in subdural haemorrhage, can be demonstrated at autopsy and affords conclusive evidence of cause of death. Rupture of tentorium has a special association with breech presentation; this is one of the main reasons why all malpresentations are excluded from consideration in this manual. Equally important, but not so well known, is the fact that virtually every case of injury to the tentorium not associated with breech presentation is associated with instrumental vaginal delivery.

There were 44 fatal cases of traumatic intracranial haemorrhage in firstborn infants delivered in the National Maternity Hospital during a period of 17 years: 27 cephalic and 17 breech presentations. All 27 cephalic presentations were delivered with forceps. There was no case of traumatic intracranial haemorrhage other than in breech or forceps delivery. This unequivocal statement is based firmly on the comprehensive postmortem coverage achieved during those years.[9]

The close correlation between trauma in the mother and trauma in the child is clearly illustrated by the 27 cases of traumatic intracranial haemorrhage in cephalic presentations described in the previous paragraph. The outcome in the 27 mothers was as follows: one death, eight blood transfusions for traumatic haemorrhage, one persistent foot-drop, and three retained in hospital for more than 2 weeks. This represents a total of 13 individuals, or almost 50%. Inexperience was not a factor in these cases: the forceps were applied by a consultant in 10, senior registrar in 14 and junior medical officer in three cases only. A clear association between trauma and duration is evident from the fact that labour was prolonged (> 12 hours) in 16 of the 27 cases.

Prevention of trauma

A sharp decline in the incidence of trauma occurred after the decision was taken to limit the duration of labour to 12 hours in the National Maternity Hospital. Meanwhile, although use of rotational forceps was discarded, no increase in the number of caesarean sections followed. The probable explanation is that more babies are born by propulsion and fewer by traction, especially combined with rotation.

An apparent anomaly in contemporary attitudes to the fetus during labour is the contrast that sometimes exists between a high level of attention paid to hypoxia and an almost casual approach to trauma. A fetus supervised with meticulous care throughout pregnancy and first stage of labour is subjected to a degree of trauma at the point of delivery which would not be considered tolerable under any circumstance a few hours later. Forcible extraction is undertaken sometimes for no better reason than that the cervix is fully dilated for a specified period. At other times trauma is inflicted in the course of a frantic effort to rescue the fetus from a condition of distress based on slender evidence. The doctor, understandably anxious to save the fetus from hypoxia, exposes it to trauma, and introduces the risk of serious injury to the mother in the process. Perinatal death in such circumstances is almost sure to be attributed to hypoxia unless an autopsy is performed, and even so it is often wrongly assumed that intracranial haemorrhage was the result of fetal distress rather than the result of treatment. The sequence of errors is complete when rupture of tentorium, which leads to intracranial haemorrhage, is attributed to cephalopelvic disproportion. Cephalopelvic disproportion is certainly not a significant factor in the aetiology of trauma in obstetrics.

Fourteen of the 27 mothers referred to above returned to the National Maternity Hospital for their second birth: 13 had a spontaneous delivery of a healthy infant, which, incidentally, weighed more than the first in 11 instances. Moreover, six of the 27 firstborn infants were preterm, thus confirming the general belief that preterm infants are more vulnerable to trauma. However, it is worthy of special note that these were the only preterm infants who died from intracranial haemorrhage in this hospital over the entire period of 17 years; all were delivered with forceps. This points to the probable conclusion that it was the forceps, not the immaturity, which was the decisive factor. Consequently, the practice of routine delivery of preterm infants with forceps is not to be recommended as a prophylactic measure against trauma.[10]

Key Points

- Trauma is associated with instrumental delivery and is therefore more common in nulliparous women
- Instrumental delivery is associated with prolonged labour
- Efficient uterine action enables a nulliparous woman to deliver herself

Pain   15

The most characteristic feature of the conventional attitude towards care in labour is the strong emphasis placed on the element of pain and, consequently, on drugs for relief of pain. Many delivery units operate from the simple premise that virtually the only, and certainly the most valuable, contribution a midwife or doctor can make to the comfort of a woman in labour is to ensure that she receives analgesic agents in adequate amounts. This passive attitude to care in labour has led to misuse of drugs; the results are far from impressive, even in the short-term sense of immediate consumer satisfaction. That there is a physical element in the discomfort of labour is not open to question, but it is equally true that the nature of the pain of labour is different from the pain associated with surgical operations or other form of injury for which similar remedies are prescribed.[10]

First stage

Pain is intermittent, lasts no longer than 1 minute, and then ceases completely. Approximately five such pains recur at regular intervals in each period of 15 minutes throughout; this amounts to a total of 100 pains during the course of a first labour of average duration. Pains occur somewhat less frequently at the beginning, and more frequently at the end. The type of pain is a cramp, comparable with primary spasmodic dysmenorrhoea, with which almost every woman is familiar.

The nature of discomfort during the first stage is quite different from the nature of discomfort during the second stage. An important component of discomfort during the first stage of labour derives from a mounting sense of frustration that a woman often endures because she feels herself to be a helpless victim of powerful natural forces, over which she can exercise little influence. Swept along on a tide of events, the purpose of which she may not fully comprehend, she tends to lose self-control. This is especially so when progress is slow and no one can say when her ordeal is likely to end. Meanwhile, attendants come and go at regular intervals of 8 hours, when for her the problem seems to begin all over again. For these particular reasons, and because of its comparatively long duration, the problem of pain in labour is essentially a problem of the first stage: the tedious hours while the cervix dilates. In this respect, yet again, a first labour is unique. Acceleration with oxytocin, therefore, can some times be more constructive than analgesia in relief of this discomfort. A dramatic improvement in the outlook of a woman in labour can be expected when the impasse which results from inefficient uterine action is broken and progress is restored – and this despite the fact that contractions are now much stronger.

Second stage

Although the physical element of discomfort is much more in evidence during the second stage of labour, a woman is generally better able to cope because she is actively engaged. Now she senses that the end is near and, moreover, that it can be hastened by her own efforts. She can regain a measure of control of the situation as the tremendous physical exertion required in pushing distracts her attention from the uterine contractions. A priori, it must be assumed that almost every woman would wish to give birth to her own child.

Reaction to pain

Women seem to react to the pain of labour in an instinctive manner: initially startled, then tense, then restive and finally limp, when with eyes tightly closed they tend to withdraw completely from contact with their surroundings. The intensity of the reaction grows with successive pains until it extends to fill the interval between contractions so that there is no longer any period of relaxation. This scenario, where a woman continues to react long after a contraction has passed, should not be allowed to develop further because contact, once lost, is seldom possible to restore. Loss of contact with a woman in labour is usually a product of poor care, to which analgesic drugs are not the appropriate response.

Surely the most impressive feature of pain in labour, however, is the extraordinary variation in the type of reaction of different individuals to what is, in effect, the same stimulus. Although objective measurements may indicate uterine contractions of similar frequency, similar strength and similar duration, the very wide range in response of different individuals affords clear evidence of the paramount importance of the subjective element in the pain of labour. Emotional stability is put to the test at times of stress, and there is no stress in the lifetime of an average person, man or woman, to compare with the birth of a first child. Hence the whole spectrum of human behaviour is revealed in a busy delivery unit in the course of a single day. To concentrate attention on the physical element of the pain of labour, to the virtual exclusion of the nature of the subjective response, is comparable to concentrating on the virulence of the organism in a case of infection, without due regard to the resistance of the host. In general terms, much more can be achieved through action taken to raise the level of resistance to stress than can be achieved by the use of analgesic drugs. This too is the humane way, because it leaves a woman in full control of her faculties, enhances her sense of dignity and permits her to give birth to her own child. In an ideal world, there would be no need for drugs at this critical juncture in one's life. In this context, the signal importance attached to duration of exposure, and to continuous personal support through labour, is discussed in Chapters 4 and 19.

Analgesia should not be given until a firm diagnosis of labour is made and, therefore, a woman is committed to delivery. This is critical, and evasions under the guise of ambivalent terms such as false or latent labour are not acceptable. The use of analgesic drugs on speculative grounds, to see what may subsequently transpire, is inappropriate. A drug given in these circumstances confuses the clinical picture for mother and staff alike. The effect is to commit the woman to delivery, even though she may not be in labour. Eventually this can result in unnecessary intervention. Whosoever administers the first drug in a delivery unit assumes a serious responsibility and should, therefore, be made acutely conscious of the possible adverse consequences of their action.

Preparation

A woman's attitude to childbirth reflects the many and varied influences to which she has been exposed since early childhood. No short-term course of lectures is likely to result in a radical change of outlook so deeply entrenched. Nevertheless, it would be difficult to exaggerate the importance attached to antenatal education in the alleviation of pain in labour in the National Maternity Hospital. The overall purpose is to convince the expectant mother that she has nothing to fear, and that she is perfectly capable of giving birth to her own child. This is subject always to two firm commitments: that duration of labour is strictly limited and that personal attention is available at all times. Consciously or otherwise, these are the two considerations that weigh most heavily on the minds of ordinary women confronted with the birth of a first child. Consequently, no effort is spared to ensure that every nulliparous woman attends these antenatal classes, on the mutual understanding that the first experience of childbirth is a matter of monumental importance to the future happiness of an entire family.

Key Points

- Relief of pain in labour is considered under four headings: antenatal education, personal attention, limited duration and analgesia

- The ability to restrict duration is crucial, because duration of exposure to stress is the dominant element in the problem of pain in labour

- Duration of labour is also crucial because it affects antenatal education, the provision of personal attention and the amount of analgesia required

Antenatal Preparation   16

Although few obstetricians, nowadays, may wish to appear openly hostile to the principle of preparation for childbirth, many continue to pay lip service only to the ideal while taking no interest whatever in the practice. This is yet another characteristic feature of the passive approach to care in labour: hopefully everything will come right on the day, and should this prove not to be the case, there are few problems not amenable to treatment with analgesia – provided enough is given and by the proper route – failing which, there is always caesarean section. This can fittingly be described as the 'less one knows the better' school of thought, which stems from lack of direct involvement in the conduct of labour.

The almost total neglect of antenatal preparation as a legitimate topic for discussion in academic circles, with the consequent lack of any authoritative guidance on organization, content or even personnel, is indicative of the state of apathy that exists within the medical establishment regarding this important subject. Physiotherapists, in particular, are left very much to themselves, suffering greatly as a consequence, both in terms of job satisfaction for the individual and professional status for the group. Direct involvement in the care in labour, on the other hand, can only lead to the conclusion that antenatal preparation is an absolutely essential element of quality care.

Purpose

The main purpose of antenatal preparation is – and should always be seen to be – to define a woman's role in labour and to teach her how to fulfil it. There are two distinct, albeit closely related, components: education and training. The educational component should seek to ensure that every expectant mother has a broad understanding of the birth process, while the training component should aim to teach her how to achieve the ultimate satisfaction of spontaneous delivery.

Practice

In the National Maternity Hospital, expectant mothers are encouraged strongly in the belief that they are well able to give birth to their own children. Thus, a spirit of self-reliance is consciously nurtured. Two firm assurances are deemed necessary: that continuous, sympathetic and informed support will be forthcoming, and that labour will not be allowed to last too long.

Content

The educational component is based on a clear description of the first and second stages of labour, couched in simple language which a lay person of reasonable intelligence can readily understand: how the first stage is concerned solely with opening of the neck of the womb, a comparatively long and tedious preliminary process over which the mother has virtually no control, and how the second stage is concerned with passage of the infant through the birth canal culminating in the actual birth, a short and somewhat turbulent process which can be brought to a rapid conclusion by the mother's own, not inconsiderable, efforts. A particular point to which great importance is attached is that everyone should be prepared for the often cataclysmic sensation of sudden pressure on the pelvic floor, which marks the transition between phase one and phase two of the second stage of labour. This is a dramatic event, which can have an altogether devastating effect when it occurs without adequate warning.

The concept of graphic representation of labour is explained in some detail, and expectant mothers are shown how this procedure is used to record rate of progress and forecast time of delivery. Everyone is given a copy of the official partogram to take away for further study, and all are expected to be familiar with the regimen when admitted eventually in labour. The simple coloured partogram, illustrated in Section II, has proved an invaluable educational instrument in this lay context.

The common forms of intervention, and the reasons for each, are explained: artificial rupture of membranes, oxytocin infusion, simple vaginal operative delivery and episiotomy. A sharp distinction is made between induction of labour and improving inefficient uterine action after labour has begun.

Pain is discussed as a subsidiary item. To place pain in its natural sequence, attention is drawn to Braxton Hicks contractions, which are very noticeable during late pregnancy, and an explanation is given for the close affinity with the contractions of uterus during labour. The effect of anxiety on the threshold for pain is frankly discussed, but care is taken not to make pain appear a central issue lest a serious disservice be done, which could indeed justify the criticism that some antenatal classes are worse than none, because women are left even more apprehensive than before. This is yet another expression of a negative, or passive, attitude towards labour.

The steps taken to supervise the welfare of the fetus are demonstrated: colour of liquor and direct auscultation as routine, extending to include electronic monitoring, scalp electrode and fetal blood sampling in particular circumstances.

Three specific items are regarded as of such outstanding practical importance that they are tested in the form of direct question and answer, as follows:

Question: How will you know when to go to hospital in labour?
Answer: When I get painful contractions which resemble period pains,

80

together with a show or persistent leakage of water – or, failing either of these, when the pains come at regular intervals of 10 minutes or less.

Question: How long will you be in hospital before your baby is born?
Answer: Six hours on average, but rarely longer than 12.
Question: Will you ever be left alone?
Answer: No.

That every woman approaching the birth of her first child should be in possession of these basic facts is considered to be the best simple assessment of the relevance of her preparation.

The training component of antenatal preparation is based on learning how to relax as the uterus contracts, during the first stage, and how to reinforce the natural expulsive forces as the head impacts on the pelvic floor, during the second phase of the second stage.

Organization

As in other areas of medical activity, careful planning can make all the difference between success and comparative failure. In the National Maternity Hospital, attention is concentrated on nulliparous women, who form a homogenous group of expectant mothers with unique problems which they approach largely with an open mind. Series of classes are confined to nulliparous women, based on the proposition that if one looks after first-time mothers well, the others will look after themselves. Parous women are segregated because, as a group, their problems are quite different; in addition, they are not infrequently prejudiced by past events. A parous woman who seeks assistance of this nature, especially for the first time, is likely to be motivated by an unfortunate previous episode. This sequence of events can have an unsettling effect on her nulliparous sisters, especially when she is anxious to recount her own experience and thus undermine the position of the teacher whenever descriptions given in class do not correspond exactly with her personal memories in every detail. Parous women tend to have closed minds on the subject of labour. They are wont to extrapolate from what is a unique occasion, in terms of individual experience, and they are frequently mistaken in the belief that others placed in a similar situation would necessarily share the same viewpoint; they do not, in a word, appreciate that women differ as much as labours differ. Courses for parous women are, therefore, held separately. Indeed, a constant theme stressed in every chapter of this manual is the need to recognize fundamental differences between nulliparous and parous women, in everything that relates to labour. Antenatal education, too, must take these differences into account.

In the case of a parous woman, the main purpose of the educator should be to convince her of the truth of the simple maxim: that a first and a subsequent labour are not in any way comparable. As this is primarily an exercise in rehabilitation, it is well to appreciate that uncritical approval of epidural anaesthesia to solve a problem that does not exist in reality, undermines a woman's confidence even further, no matter how grateful she may appear to be.

In the National Maternity Hospital, classes are arranged to correspond with antenatal clinics, so that it is possible to attend both at the same visit with the minimum of inconvenience. There are 13 courses running each week, nine of which include partners with two classes in the evening. There are only two courses for parous women. The course begins at 30 weeks of pregnancy so that the recently acquired knowledge may remain fresh in mind. Discussion is encouraged, but much time is saved by anticipating the questions that are sure to be asked. Six sessions of 1 hour are devoted to labour. The number of classes is purposely restricted because as classes increase in number so do defaulters. Limiting the number of classes also helps concentrate the attention of both audience and teacher, and thus reduces the tendency to boredom. Three classes are devoted to an understanding of the physical process of childbirth and three classes to the practice of relaxation and propulsion, at the appropriate stages. A video is shown at which husbands are welcome. Finally, there is a conducted tour of the delivery unit. Almost 80% of nulliparous women avail of the complete package.

Personnel

To achieve its full potential, antenatal education must be conducted under enlightened supervision, to ensure that the efforts of the educators are coordinated and that the content is relevant to clinical practice in the particular institution. This presumes that clinical practice is consistent, otherwise it is difficult to imagine how the educators can function effectively. Individual educators should be midwives or physiotherapists who have ongoing practical experience in the delivery unit in question. These two disciplines correspond broadly with the educational and training components previously mentioned. No educator should be engaged exclusively in this area because this inevitably leads to a condition of isolation, which is one of the main factors militating against proper recognition of educational programmes of this nature.

As mutual confidence is the keynote, this requires that educators appear to know precisely what they are talking about in strictly technical terms, and in relation to actual practice in the particular institution. Naturally, they should also have insight into the anxieties peculiar to a group of women faced with the challenge of a lifetime. Incidentally, educators should be acutely conscious of the exceptional opportunity afforded them to provide a favourable image of the entire maternity service to the consumers. Too often educators and practitioners appear to be almost in direct conflict with each other, because they have developed little or no common ground.

Key Points

- Antenatal education deserves much more attention than it currently receives
- The development of antenatal education to reflect consistent practice in the supervision of labour would be of enormous benefit

Analgesic Drugs   17

Pethidine

Pethidine is the standard drug for relief of pain in labour. Although far from ideal for the purpose, no drug has yet emerged to seriously challenge pethidine. The reason is that the power of a drug to relieve pain is in direct proportion to its potential adverse effects.

Disadvantages of pethidine

Pethidine has many disadvantages that are wholly unpredictable in individual cases. Some women suffer from intractable nausea and vomiting, sufficient to turn childbirth into a miserable experience. Some become profoundly depressed, introspective, and so overwhelmed with self-pity that they lapse eventually into a state of stupor, from which they are roused only by contractions to make aimless protests and demand more and more drugs, until the original situation is compounded and a vicious circle is established. Some become completely disorientated and so confused that they are quite unable to cooperate with their attendants, especially during the second stage of labour, when cooperation is essential if spontaneous delivery is to be achieved.

The most serious possible adverse effect of pethidine is on the child. Depression of the respiratory centre may delay the establishment of normal breathing in the critical minutes after birth.

The question remains whether the advantages of pethidine are outweighed by the disadvantages, to the extent that the use of pethidine in labour should be discontinued completely. The truth is that it is simply not possible to provide sufficient pethidine to relieve pain in labour effectively without introducing an extraneous element of discomfort and, sometimes, danger. The problem is that there is no more suitable drug available. Relief of pain in labour, therefore, must of necessity entail a genuine compromise between a reasonable degree of analgesia and a reasonable element of iatrogenic discomfort in the case of the mother, with possible depression of the nervous system in the case of the child.

A number of drugs have been recommended in combination with pethidine, in the hope that they might enhance the desirable effects or neutralize the undesirable. None has proved successful. As a matter of medical principle, drugs in combination are best avoided – they cross the placenta, may confuse the diagnosis of fetal distress and can cause problems in the newborn which endure for a considerable time: diazepam, which can be detected weeks later, is a classic example.

Naloxone is a specific opiate antagonist and should be instantly available whenever pethidine is used.

Use of pethidine

Pethidine should not be used on a routine basis simply to comply with some obstetric ritual, or to protect staff from possible criticism later. An obstetrician who appears critical of a midwife because an occasional woman subsequently complains that she has not had sufficient pain relief, encourages this form of mass medication. Doctors are seldom present to witness the particular circumstances and it is all too easy for them to pose as being more humane, after the event. No personal commitment is required for this mode of behaviour. The strongest arguments in favour of large doses of analgesic drugs during labour are advanced mostly by obstetricians who do not themselves spend much time in a delivery unit. Pethidine, it must be strongly emphasized, often makes labour more unpleasant than it otherwise would have been; moreover, the more pethidine a woman receives, the more disgruntled she often becomes. Indeed, the woman who complains most vehemently, both during and after the event, is not infrequently herself the victim of a surfeit of drugs.

The practice with Active Management of Labour is to await the reaction of every woman to her unique personal experience of labour. Each woman is cared for as an individual in this respect. Expectant mothers are advised that all methods of pain relief are available, but that prior commitments are not given because this is considered not to serve the best interests of the individual. Expectant mothers are, however, given a firm assurance that the duration of exposure will be strictly limited and that a personal nurse will be present at all times. They are, in other words, encouraged to consider the problem of pain relief in a wider context.

First stage

Pethidine is given only with the informed consent of the mother, and only during the first stage of labour. A small dose is preferred initially because, should a large dose be given and side effects follow, the error cannot so easily be rectified. Additional injections are given if the desired effect is not achieved and side effects are not troublesome. Epidural anaesthesia is considered if no relief of pain is achieved or side effects are a problem. Strict control over the use of analgesic agents fosters a more constructive approach to the overall problem of stress in labour.

Second stage

There is not nearly the same need for analgesia during the second stage of labour, because during contractions mothers are usually preoccupied with the immediate task in hand. This distraction operates as a most effective method of pain relief. Properly harnessed, this sense of active participation can alter the whole outlook.

Inhalation analgesia in the form of nitrous oxide, which is self-administered, is generally confined to the latter part of phase two of the second stage of labour, and is used, therefore, for a relatively short period; prolonged exposure to nitrous oxide may result in hyperventilation with alkalosis and dehydration, apart from a severe hangover. During the hectic moments, as the head crowns, the benefit that accrues from this form of analgesia seems to derive at least as much from the inducement to breathe in and out, rather than push, as from the direct effect of the gas itself.

Ventouse delivery usually requires local infiltration of the perineum only. Simple forceps delivery is conducted under pudendal block if there is no epidural anaesthesia in place. Rotation with forceps is not performed in the National Maternity Hospital.

Key Points

- There is no ideal drug for relief of pain in labour
- No drug whatsoever should be given before a firm diagnosis of labour is made and the woman, therefore, is committed to delivery

Epidural Anaesthesia   18

Epidural anaesthesia provides almost complete relief of pain and is not associated with any of the unpleasant side effects of pethidine. The mother retains her mental acuity and the infant is alert at birth. There are few more impressive sights than the resolution of maternal distress which follows successful epidural anaesthesia. The answer to the problem of maternal stress in labour might, therefore, appear simple: make epidural anaesthesia available on a comprehensive scale and encourage everyone to avail of the service. However, this would be a gross oversimplification of a much more complex problem because, although epidural anaesthesia is far more effective than pethidine, it too can have adverse effects.

Direct adverse effects

The most serious direct adverse effect of epidural analgesia is accidental entry of the anaesthetic agent into the cerebrospinal fluid; although rare, this can have significant and sometimes serious sequelae. Other less serious direct adverse effects include loss of mobility, retention of urine, inefficient uterine action and abnormalities in the fetal heart rate, sometimes resulting in unnecessary caesarean section. Like any other procedure careful audit must be maintained.

Indirect adverse effects

The indirect adverse effects of epidural anaesthesia are an aspect of labour to which far too little attention is paid. The procedure can affect important decisions in management and will increase the workload of the midwife.

Sometimes epidural anaesthesia is given before a firm diagnosis of labour is established. The result is that, after much confusion, a caesarean section is eventually performed on a woman who was not in labour. An epidural should not be given until a diagnosis of labour is firmly established and the woman is, therefore, committed to delivery.

Epidural anaesthesia is sometimes used as a palliative procedure when labour is prolonged, as if duration of itself were not important, provided the mother suffers no pain. This approach to the subject of pain illustrates the fundamental difference between the philosophies that underlie active and passive management of labour. Active Management of Labour is based on the proposition that the risks increase proportionately with the duration of labour, whether or not a woman suffers pain. Indeed, total relief of pain can create a sense of false security when labour is prolonged. Rupture of uterus is the ultimate expression of trauma in the mother, and epidural anaesthesia has emerged as an important factor in the aetiology of this calamity in recent years. The strongest possible recommendation is that epidural anaesthesia should not be used as a substitute for corrective action in cases of prolonged labour, especially in parous women.

Epidural anaesthesia may result in an increase in the number of operative deliveries if efficient uterine action is reduced. However, the number of spontaneous deliveries can be increased significantly when there is the will to do so.[11] Motivation to this end depends largely on a clear appreciation of the importance of mothers giving birth to their own children. The solution, as with so much else in labour, depends on ensuring efficient uterine action. Previous chapters have dealt with how to ensure efficient uterine action during the first stage of labour. Care in the second stage of labour is altered if the urge to push is removed. Improved methods of administration with continuous infusion of low concentration of anaesthetic agent can also diminish this problem.

In the absence of an urge to push on diagnosis of full dilatation, and with the fetal head high in the pelvis and the occiput in the transverse position, 1 hour is allowed to pass before pelvic examination is repeated. Then, if the head has descended to the level of the pelvic floor, pushing is encouraged. Oxytocin may be started if subsequent progress is poor.

If, after 1 hour, the head has not descended to the level of the pelvic floor, oxytocin is started and pelvic examination is repeated after a further hour. Pushing is then commenced for 1 hour and, if delivery is not imminent, pelvic examination is performed with a view to a simple vaginal operative delivery.

Case selection

There is a need to define a joint midwifery and medical approach to epidural anaesthesia.

The first conclusion is that epidural anaesthesia has an invaluable contribution to make to labour in nulliparous women, but, equally important, that the relative contribution to labour in parous women is much less. High use of epidural anaesthesia in parous women stems from the mistaken belief that a valid comparison can be drawn between a first and a subsequent labour. A woman who has had an unpleasant first experience, during which she may or may not have had epidural anaesthesia, frequently seeks a prior commitment on the next occasion because she fears that the experience is likely to be repeated. There are no grounds for this misapprehension. Obstetricians would serve the interests of the parous woman better were they to dispel her fears with a simple explanation of the essential difference between a first and a second birth. Moreover, it is in parous women that epidural anaesthesia acts to increase the risk of ruptured uterus, partly because the parous uterus is prone to rupture, and partly because pain has an important warning function in this regard.

The second conclusion is that it is unwise to enter into a prior commitment, even with a nulliparous woman. There are two sound reasons why an expectant approach to epidural anaesthesia should be practised: the reaction of each individual to the actual experience of first labour can rarely be foretold, perhaps least of all by the woman herself; and the duration of first labour cannot be predicted.

Subject to the above reservations, women who derive most benefit from epidural anaesthesia fall into three broad groups, as follows:

- those who are so disturbed at the very prospect of labour that they are already unduly upset at the point of admission
- those who, despite an initial appearance of composure, become unduly upset soon afterwards
- those who are not in sight of delivery after 6 hours.

The number in the first group is related closely to antenatal preparation, the number in the second group to the quality of care after admission, and the number in the third group to the duration of labour.

Responsibility

Professional responsibility for epidural anaesthesia deserves attention, especially where a prior commitment has been made, or where the person involved is a parous woman.

Can it be presumed that the mother, in requesting epidural anaesthesia, gives blanket acceptance to all the consequences, direct and indirect, without being in a position to fully understand? And how far does an obstetrician meet the professional obligation by sanctioning a procedure several months in advance and, therefore, without due regard to the particular circumstances at the time of administration? And what of the anaesthetist summoned to provide an emergency service with little or no knowledge of the background, obstetric or otherwise? Finally, and because timing is crucial, there is the midwife whose decision may be of vital importance, particularly in the case of a parous woman. These issues do not arise when the decision to use epidural anaesthesia is made on a selective basis during the course of labour.

Key Points

- Epidural anaesthesia has a special contribution to make to labour management in nulliparous women
- Epidural anaesthesia must be treated with caution, especially in parous women
- The outcome of labour in relation to epidural anaesthesia must be carefully audited
- Epidural anaesthesia should not be used as a cover for prolonged labour
- Efficient uterine action remains the key to normality

Personal Attention   19

One of the most disturbing prospects of labour is fear of isolation, which the mere mention of a delivery unit seems to engender in many women. This fear of isolation is certainly not a reflection on the standard of medical practice as ordinarily understood; quite the contrary, the problem tends to increase as technical standards rise. The more efficient a unit in strictly medical terms, the more isolated the mothers are likely to feel. The result is that the average person seems to have reached the conclusion that medical efficiency and humane considerations are just not compatible.

Moral support

Childbirth is a unique event which should provide a sense of profound and lasting satisfaction for mothers, and in which midwives and doctors could count themselves fortunate to share. Yet there are many women who complain bitterly of the apparent indifference of those in whom they placed their trust during the most vulnerable period of their lives. Those closest to the action often do not appear to realize that there are few places on this earth so lonely as a busy delivery unit. As human consciousness is seldom more open to impression than during the momentous hours of labour, a casual approach to yet another routine assignment may leave a mother with a burning sense of resentment. Apparently trivial episodes such as curt tone of voice, bloodstained glove, mindless exposure in the indelicate lithotomy position or failure to convey the result of vaginal examination, though not seemingly of great consequence in themselves, still portray an often deplorable lack of sensitivity in professional staff who should know a great deal better. Because of the heightened sense of awareness at this time, the memory of these affronts to their personal dignity, unintentional though they may be, are nonetheless preserved indefinitely, and in photographic detail, by many women.

The steady emotional decline that is a characteristic feature of labour not properly supervised follows an entirely predictable course. The scenario can be written beforehand. The woman becomes progressively withdrawn from contact with her environment, closes her eyes and buries her face in the pillow, only later to become increasingly restive, with contorted features and aimless movements interrupted by frantic outbursts, until eventually a state of panic is reached and self-control is lost completely. Once the morale of a woman in labour has begun to crumble, it becomes more and more difficult to restore the balance. Midwives, particularly, must be acutely conscious of the need to keep every woman in labour on a tight emotional rein from the point of admission until her baby is born, because the further she is allowed to slip down the emotional incline, the more difficult it becomes to recover her composure. Specifically, women in labour must be encouraged to keep their eyes open at all times; closed eyes usually mark the first step along the road to disintegration. The best protection possible against the gradual erosion of a woman's personal dignity in labour is to hold her attention firmly from the outset.

A sense of panic is a shattering experience from which the individual may never fully recover. This may lead to recurrent nightmares, permanent revulsion to childbirth with consequent marital disharmony, and a sense of antagonism even towards her own child. Not nearly enough attention is paid to this aspect of trauma in childbirth. Panic should rank as one of the most serious complications in obstetrics – more serious than ruptured uterus, in many respects – and it should never be allowed to happen. Much less serious emotional disturbance than this has caused some, albeit misguided, women to advocate a return to home confinement, while freely acknowledging that the purely medical case in favour of hospital confinement remains overwhelming. Consequently, there is a pressing need to recognize that a morbid fear of isolation during labour is widespread, to acknowledge that this fear is only too well founded in practice and to resolve that effective action must be taken to rectify the unfortunate situation.

The midwife

The only effective antidote to the dread of isolation is a prior guarantee to every expectant mother of continuous personal attention through labour. Personal attention, in this context, means one midwife to one woman, face to face. What personal attention does *not* mean is a group of nurses caring for an equivalent number of patients on a collective basis. Although the total complement of nursing staff deployed in a particular delivery unit may be more than adequate on paper, many women continue to complain of being left alone for comparatively long periods. Positive steps are necessary, therefore, to ensure that each woman in labour identifies, by name, with an individual midwife. Although the physical presence of a trained companion is, in itself, a source of considerable comfort to a woman in labour, mere physical presence is not nearly enough. The midwife must appreciate that her primary duty to the mother is to provide the emotional support so desperately needed at this critical time; it is not simply to monitor vital signs in a detached clinical manner. The physical condition of the mother must, of course, be supervised, but this is just a matter of recording a few basic items at regular intervals of, say, 2 hours. These conventional record systems have very little relevance to the great majority of healthy women who are delivered within a few hours of admission. In many centres an altogether disproportionate amount of space on the partogram is allotted to such observations, seemingly to allow for the possibility that every woman might develop fulminating eclampsia or continue in labour for at least 24 hours!

The real value of a personal midwife is best reflected in the facial expression of a woman in labour. Each midwife must purposefully strive to establish a genuine sense of rapport with her charge by seeking to identify everyday topics of common interest. By far the most impressive evidence of the quality of care afforded in a delivery unit is to observe midwife and mother engaged in animated conversation, exchanging smiles in the process. Smiles are more effective than drugs as an antidote to pain. Some are clearly better than others in the field of human relationships, but almost anyone can become proficient when they are trained to be sufficiently aware of the need. A woman's experience of labour depends to a very great extent on the quality of the relationship established with her personal midwife.

The midwife, for her part, derives her greatest satisfaction from the opportunity to contribute so much to one under such stress. Those who share moments of great stress tend to forge a lasting bond, and it is truly remarkable how often a woman can recall an individual midwife by name, and her kindness, many years after her first confinement. Naturally, communication at this level is much easier to establish in the context of a common culture. Although it is likely to be more difficult when the cultural background of the midwife differs widely from that of her charge, failure to communicate, in any meaningful sense of the word, arises much more often from the midwife not having been taught to appreciate the need. Specifically, every midwife has a responsibility to ensure that the mother genuinely understands the purpose of each intervention and the result of each examination, and that she is kept informed of current progress, with a regular review of the time at which her baby is expected to be born.

A prior guarantee is given to every expectant mother who attends the National Maternity Hospital that she will have a personal midwife through the whole of labour, from the point of admission until her baby is born, without regard to the hour of day or night. Many mothers, and observers too, believe this to be the most important development in the care of labour in recent years, but they do not always realize that it would not be feasible unless the duration of labour was restricted. The authors rate personal attention as second only in importance to limitation of duration in the care of labour, although the two items are inseparable since one cannot be achieved without the other. With almost 8000 deliveries per annum, the provision of a personal midwife for every woman in labour is no mean achievement.

The doctor

Doctors must recognize that they too have an indispensable role to play in the provision of personalized care and attention, which is a central issue in good care in labour. The consultant obstetrician, who is ultimately responsible for the welfare of all mothers, must set a clear example because, inevitably, the attitude of the consultant pervades the entire system. Young midwives and doctors follow the example set by their teachers. Unfortunately, on attainment of consultant status, many obstetricians virtually abandon the delivery unit for the antenatal ward or, more likely, the operating theatre, and henceforth, in so far as labour is concerned, their attention is confined to a small cohort of abnormal cases. Even senior registrars are seldom seen in some delivery units until the need for surgical intervention arises. The result is that care in labour in normal women, who represent the overwhelming majority in any given unit, is left to junior residents who have far less experience than senior midwives.

There is absolutely no point in consultant obstetricians advocating a standard of care and attention to which they are not prepared to make a positive contribution: they must be seen to practise what they preach. This means that consultants must be seen in the delivery unit at frequent intervals every day, and they must discuss directly with each expectant mother the questions that they should know to be uppermost in her mind on this momentous occasion. Consultants, in other words, must underwrite the whole ethos of care in labour by personal example.

The husband

The extent to which husbands should be influenced to remain with their wives during the entire course of labour and delivery remains an open question. Sometimes it is difficult to avoid the impression that husbands are enlisted to protect their wives against the fear of isolation which is the subject matter of the present chapter, and sometimes, even, to protect them from unwarranted intervention. Experience suggests that women have far more to gain from the presence of a female companion who is not only sympathetic but also well informed and, therefore, in a much better position to provide the type of firm support and guidance so sorely needed.

Key Points

- Continual personal attention is an indicator of the quality of care afforded in any delivery unit
- Mothers regard continual personal attention as the most important contribution to care in labour
- The ability to provide continual personal attention is closely related to duration of labour

Role of Doctor   20

The role of the doctor in supervision of labour needs to be considered at four quite different levels of responsibility.

Consultant obstetricians

Consultant obstetricians are in a unique position to influence the standard of care in labour for the better, simply by agreeing a common policy within the confines of each institution. The main obstacle to improvement in the quality of care in labour in most institutions is lack of clear direction from the top. Midwives and resident medical officers are frequently placed in the invidious position of having to apply different methods of care, in exactly the same clinical circumstances, for no reason other than that the names of the consultants printed on the charts are different. A good illustration of this anomaly is when patients in adjacent beds receive different concentrations of oxytocin or different analgesic drugs, for no more convincing reason than that they happen to have attended the antenatal clinic on different days. The sheer irrationality of this mode of action is a constant affront to the intelligence of professional staff. No one would dare suggest that an intensive care unit in a general hospital could operate efficiently under direction of such a capricious nature. Hence, wherever a genuine wish to improve the quality of care afforded to women in labour exists, the first essential requirement is for the consultant obstetricians to come together and agree to surrender a small portion of their jealously guarded independence for the sake of the common good. This, the authors suggest, is the acid test of goodwill at consultant level. Without this degree of cooperation a delivery unit cannot even begin to achieve its full potential. Naturally, someone must be prepared to take the initial step.

First, a chain of command must be sharply defined. There should be one person only in charge of a delivery unit at any given time; a delivery unit cannot operate efficiently under a committee system. For practical purposes the person responsible must be a midwife. She should be designated as Midwife-in-Charge, or Sister, and wear a distinctive uniform that can be recognized instantly by all concerned. Everyone who works in the unit should be subject to her immediate authority. There is no more room for divided responsibility in a delivery unit than there is aboard a ship at sea.

Next, the most sensitive areas of care must be clearly identified and the general outline of procedure standardized. These matters have been addressed in previous chapters under the appropriate headings, as follows: diagnosis, progress, duration, acceleration, etc.

After the critical decision to delegate authority, the most valuable contribution the consultant can make to care in labour is to fully accept responsibility for the outcome. There is no place for equivocation on this issue; delegation of authority on any other basis is meaningless. A bland declaration to the general effect is worthless; subordinate staff need to be convinced that no scapegoat will be sought whenever a mishap occurs – as sooner or later it undoubtedly will as long as humans remain fallible. In practice, unfortunately, this is too often the case: wherever there is a lack of trust, decisions are avoided, care is not pursued effectively and caesarean sections are performed unnecessarily because surgery provides a soft option for those anxious to avoid blame. Contrary to superficial appearances, the decision to commit a woman to caesarean section is taken usually by resident staff before the consultant, who may eventually perform the operation, is even notified.

Consultant obstetricians should be at pains to show equal concern for the composure of all women in labour, and not concentrate his attention on the few who are abnormal. They should be ever conscious of the potential to boost morale by frequent appearances on the 'shop floor'. However, they should not interfere officiously in routine matters, but rather encourage staff to get on with the good work themselves.

The Mastership system, where one individual bears the ultimate responsibility for all mothers and babies for a maximum period of 7 years, is a distinctive feature of all the Dublin Maternity Hospitals; it facilitates a high level of cooperation amongst professional colleagues.

Senior residents

Senior residents working in the National Maternity Hospital must hold a specialist qualification in obstetrics and gynaecology: there is a strict rule that one must be instantly available, on the premises, at all times. The most important function of the senior resident is to review the condition of every woman in the delivery unit at regular intervals of 4 hours approximately, especially late at night. The senior resident is expected to be on familiar terms with every woman in labour and not, as frequently happens, to remain aloof until summoned to undertake an operative delivery. All but a few obstetric cases are normal at the point of admission, yet many more become abnormal subsequently, simply because they are not supervised properly from the outset. Most complications of labour develop in hospital, and could be readily avoided if proper care and attention commenced at the time of admission. The primary duty of the senior resident is to ensure that this simple proposition is put into daily practice. A good personal relationship with the midwife in charge is an essential prerequisite to achieving this end.

The senior resident, in consultation always with the midwife in charge, decides when to intervene and chooses the method of delivery, except in the case of caesarean section which must be referred to the consultant. The need to intervene on the conventional grounds of failure to advance, or maternal distress, declines sharply when a policy of active participation is pursued from the beginning. The only operative methods of delivery now practised in the National Maternity Hospital are caesarean section or low forceps and ventouse deliveries. There is no opportunity for trainee specialists to acquire what some might still regard as an essential skill, like forceps rotation, because this, as other manoeuvres, is no longer practised. Nowadays, senior residents are cast firmly in the role of obstetric physicians, rather than surgeons, with most emphasis on supervision of labour in normal cases.

Residents

Resident medical officers working in the National Maternity Hospital are in a position of training, either as specialists or family practitioners. None is involved directly in the decision-making process. Residents are cast in the role of graduate students whose main purpose is to learn about normal birth; it is assuredly not to teach others how to solve complicated clinical problems of which they themselves have little or no experience. Most young doctors are only too relieved when this situation is frankly acknowledged, because no intelligent young man or woman would wish to be placed in a false position where it is necessary to pretend a level of expertise which they, and indeed everyone else, knows they do not possess. Those who do not readily accept this position represent a potential hazard to all concerned. Although a resident is on duty in the delivery unit of the National Maternity Hospital at all times – a practical advantage of scale – this is not considered a necessary feature of good practice. Residents are always subject to the authority of the midwife in charge and function entirely under her supervision. Practical tasks performed by residents are: artificial rupture of membranes, low forceps or ventouse deliveries and perineal repair. The midwife in charge consults directly with the senior registrar whenever she is in doubt about the care of an individual case. The resident is never in a position to dictate to the midwife, nor to overrule her decision in any matter whatsoever.

Medical students

Clinical obstetrics is presented to undergraduates in a manner quite different from previous years. Nowadays the aim is purely educational. Undergraduate teaching is based on the assumption that all births take place in hospital, and that comparatively few doctors, therefore, will ever again attend a woman in labour. Nevertheless, it is considered to be one of the fundamental requirements of medical education, in the broadest sense, that every doctor, no matter what discipline may be pursued in later life, should observe at close quarters the nature of childbirth and understand the implications of current care in labour. With this in mind, every medical student must complete 8 hours on 7 consecutive days in the delivery unit, providing continuous personal attention for one mother each day, in a face-to-face relationship. A medical student must function alone, and one student only is permitted in the delivery unit at any given time. Medical students are subject to the same discipline as student midwives. A medical student is not permitted to leave a woman in labour without the express permission of the midwife in charge, and then only when a replacement is immediately available. At the end of 7 days the medical student must submit a written report on seven labours conducted under personal supervision, devoting special attention to the emotional impact on the mother, which the student has shared.

A medical student may not leave a woman in labour to observe an operative, twin or breech delivery, even when conducted in an adjoining room. The student is given clearly to understand that the commitment to a woman in labour must be absolute, and that it is the very negation of good obstetric teaching to make use of a woman in labour for one's own advantage, only to abandon her when something more spectacular comes along. This is usually the first, and probably the last, occasion in the whole medical curriculum on which a student comes face to face with a person under severe emotional stress for an extended period of time; it is a salutary experience, one that can be turned to good effect in other branches of medicine. Medical students are immensely gratified to find how much they can contribute by personal commitment in these circumstances. This close encounter with individuals under stress is regarded as the essence of undergraduate education on the subject of labour. No longer are medical students exposed to obstetrical curiosities and complicated deliveries: the emphasis is placed on normal birth. It is seen as no function of undergraduate teaching to produce a doctor qualified to commence practice in obstetrics on the day after graduation. A future family practitioner, who may wish to provide antenatal and postnatal care in conjunction with a specialist unit, is required to serve 6 months as a junior resident in obstetrics after graduation.

Key Points

- Consultant obstetricians who cannot agree a common overall policy arguably represent the main impediment to improving the standard of care in a labour ward

- One consultant should have overall responsibility for the labour ward

- The role of junior resident medical staff should be redefined as graduate student

- The attention of undergraduates should be directed towards the emotional impact of labour rather than to technical procedures

Role of Midwife 21

The role of the midwife in the care of labour is considered at three levels in the National Maternity Hospital. A Sister, or Midwife-in-Charge, and a staff midwife are both state registered general nurses and trained midwives, at different levels of experience. A student midwife is likewise a state registered nurse, having completed 3 years of vocational training in an accredited general hospital and passed a public examination. Midwifery is a postgraduate subject that requires 2 additional years of specialist experience and a similar examination.

Sister-in-Charge

The Sister is of paramount importance and it is openly acknowledged that hers is a vital role. In practice she must make all the critical decisions which otherwise could go by default: she must confirm or reject the diagnosis of labour in every case admitted; she must measure dilatation of cervix at regular intervals; she must decide when to accelerate progress; and she must carry these decisions into effect – day and night – without reference to medical staff who may be otherwise engaged, if not asleep in bed. Finally, she must decide when the limits of her authority are reached and seek consultation. All this adds up to a formidable responsibility, which requires strength of character as well as years of clinical experience.

Whenever the Sister decides that the limits of her authority are reached, the opportunity for consultation with a medical colleague of comparable status is always readily available. It would seem utterly incongruous if a fellow professional with such wide experience of a highly specialized nature were placed in the position of having to seek the advice of a junior resident with a primary medical qualification. The practical exposure of the average junior resident is restricted to hasty appearances at normal births during a short period of undergraduate residence, possibly instructed by the self-same midwife.

The Sister in the delivery unit of the National Maternity Hospital is vested with the authority necessary to perform the duties of her office effectively. Specifically, she does not consult with any doctor below the status of senior registrar. As each Sister is personally responsible for some 1500 deliveries per annum, she is recognized as an expert in the field, and her advice is keenly sought by members of the medical staff at every level, and on all aspects of labour.

The influence of the Sister is no less important at a humane level. An air of quiet efficiency, which is the hallmark of a good delivery unit, depends on her. This intangible element, which communicates itself so easily to a sensitive observer, is an essential ingredient of the spirit of mutual trust that is such a necessary component of good care. Mothers need to sense that the midwives and doctors to whose care they are committed during these difficult hours behave as members of a team, each with a known part to play. As captain of the team, no one compares with the Sister, so she surely has the right to expect the unqualified support of colleagues – doctors as well as midwives – in her onerous task. A delivery unit cannot begin to function smoothly without a developed team spirit; everyone suffers when this is lacking.

Five senior midwives with the rank of Sister are employed in the delivery unit of the National Maternity Hospital. There is always one on duty, day and night, and only one, to guard against the possible adverse effects of division of responsibility. The actual hours worked are flexible; these are left largely as a matter of mutual agreement. There is no permanent night duty. The Sister devotes her undivided attention to women in labour. There are no other duties to be performed. She is not responsible for a hospital ward, nor for an operating theatre in the event of caesarean section. She wears a distinctive uniform so that she can be recognized instantly. Without a doubt, her greatest reward is the tremendous sense of job satisfaction that derives from the ability to make such a worthwhile contribution to the resolution of the perennial problem of stress in labour, on what truly could be described as a grand scale. Among the many benefits that have accrued from the practice of Active Management of Labour, none is more gratifying to observe than the boost given to the professional status of midwives in this hospital.

Staff midwife

A staff midwife acts as personal assistant to the Sister and is responsible directly to her. Two senior staff midwives are present at all times and their hours of duty correspond with those of the Sister. A senior staff midwife, like Sister, acts mainly in a supervisory capacity and in normal circumstances is not identified with an individual mother. At least one staff midwife is present at every delivery, and most deliveries are conducted without reference to medical staff.

Two junior staff midwives make up the complement. They are trained midwives who are practising under direct supervision by the Sister.

Student midwife

Four student midwives complete a team. A student midwife plays a different role. She provides continuous support for one woman through labour. The role ensures that she soon comes to appreciate that a midwife's unique contribution to the conduct of labour is made at a personal level. This requires that far more attention be paid to a woman's face than to her abdomen, or to her vital signs. As this is a midwifery training school, students perform these duties under constant supervision; they would be suitable for trained personnel otherwise.

The procedure is as follows: the mother is admitted to the delivery unit by a student midwife who remains with her during labour, carries out the delivery, presents her newborn infant and, eventually, accompanies her to the postnatal ward. This ideal is not always realized fully because it is affected by hours of duty, but as labour rarely lasts longer than 8 hours it applies in most cases. It is very seldom that more than two midwives are involved, consecutively, with the same woman. Each student midwife keenly appreciates that her primary duty is to sustain her charge's flagging spirits during the tedious hours of the first stage, and then to encourage her to achieve spontaneous delivery through her own efforts in the second stage. Student midwives spend 6 months, out of the total period of 2 years required for midwifery training, in the delivery unit.

General principles

The personal midwife is instructed to sit always in front of, and in direct eye contact with, a recumbent mother. She must not stand over her, in a dominant position, and never behind, out of her line of vision. A comfortable seat is provided for this purpose. Should a woman prefer to walk, her midwife accompanies her.

Midwives are encouraged to develop close personal relationships with mothers, and to converse with them freely on any subject which holds their interest, thus distracting attention from the labour predicament. In our experience, young, properly motivated women perform this task with remarkable success when they are made sufficiently conscious of the need, and given the right example by their superiors. Midwives are taught that women in labour have a natural tendency to withdraw from contact with their surroundings and turn inwards on themselves, and that this inclination to introspection is exaggerated greatly by analgesic drugs. They are forewarned about the woman who closes her eyes, buries her face in the pillow and continues to complain even between contractions. They know that these are signs which indicate that the thread of personal contact is being eroded and that, once broken, it will be very difficult to mend. They are acutely sensitive to the fact that a woman who turns her back is passing a devastating judgement on the quality of the midwifery care.

The two subjects of conversation that are of abiding interest to a woman in labour are the expected time of delivery and the welfare of her unborn child. A good midwife appreciates the need for constant reassurance that steady progress is being made and that the baby is likely to be born soon. This information should be instantly demonstrable on any worthwhile partogram. Hopefully, the partogram will have been thoroughly explained beforehand, at antenatal classes, with this important sequel in mind. In that case, mothers can be expected to take a keen interest in the proceedings. A partogram that does not fulfil this simple predictive function has forfeited much of its value.

Specific duties

The personal midwife has specific clinical duties to perform at regular intervals during labour. She must record the mother's pulse, temperature, respirations, blood pressure and urine, as well as the fetal heart and liquor. In the event of oxytocin being used, she must regulate the rate of infusion and enter each contraction as it occurs. As a student, she works under close supervision and must report any untoward event to her immediate superior.

Key Points

- Care in labour cannot be effective unless organization of the delivery unit is the responsibility of a designated midwife

- Mutual confidence must exist between midwives and doctors at every level

- A clear chain of command must be in place

- Midwives and doctors should appreciate that much more can be contributed to emotional equilibrium than to physical survival in circumstances where most maternity cases are normal at the point of admission

Role of Mother   **22**

It could too easily be overlooked that mothers themselves have the most important contribution of all to make to the birth process. No matter how high the quality of care on offer from midwives and doctors, the entire experience may well prove disastrous when the mother is not properly prepared. Therefore, a serious obligation rests on expectant mothers to take full advantage of the educational facilities available, so as to learn the nature of their role and how best this can be fulfilled. Mothers should not be allowed – any more than midwives or doctors are allowed – to evade their responsibilities in this matter. They should be disabused of the notion that midwives and doctors can be expected to cope with the inevitable turmoil as part of their normal duties. Paternalism is not to be considered a virtue here; an expectant mother should be made to face the fact that the birth of her child is primarily her responsibility.

All this is to presume that adequate educational facilities are both readily available and relevant in content. First and foremost, what is taught must be seen to correspond directly with everyday practice in the institution. It is not just teachers who must be credible; midwives and doctors also must know exactly what women have been taught to expect, prior to admission. If more than lip service is to be paid to the proposition that education is a necessary component of an obstetric service with pretensions to optimal standards of care in labour, then classes must cease to be regarded as optional extras, conducted by teachers who are far removed from clinical practice and virtually ignored by those in positions of greatest influence. The most important element in the entire educational process is, of course, education to the need for education: only clinicians are in a position to impress this on their charges. It is much too late to begin education in a labour ward.

Every adult woman must, in the final analysis, be made to feel the proper custodian of her personal well-being, not to mention that of her child. Labour is no exception to this general rule. An expectant mother owes it to herself, her husband and her child, and to every other woman sharing the facilities of the same delivery unit, to be well briefed on the subject of a mother's contribution to labour. The disruptive effect of one disorganized and frightened woman in a delivery unit extends far beyond her individual comfort and safety, and there should be no hesitation in telling her so.

Mothers also have a duty to those who care for them during labour. The reciprocal nature of this compact deserves much more emphasis than it is given.

Where necessary, it should be bluntly stated that midwives are not expected to submit themselves to the sometimes outrageous conduct of perfectly healthy women who cannot be persuaded to cross a narrow corridor from an antenatal clinic to attend classes. Such women must learn how to behave with dignity and purpose during the most important event of their lives. Nor should midwives be held responsible for the degrading scenes that occasionally result from failure of a woman to fulfil her part of the compact.

Women who have participated in the educational programme at the National Maternity Hospital generally portray a high level of insight into the essential features of the birth process. They understand the need for professional confirmation of their provisional diagnosis of labour, they know that subsequent progress is measured in terms of opening of the neck of the womb and, when progress is slow, they appreciate that it makes good sense to take corrective action at the proper time. All this is evident from the partogram with which they are already familiar. It is hardly surprising, therefore, that women in labour often request acceleration with oxytocin when it becomes clear that satisfactory progress is not being made. By way of contrast, they need to be convinced whenever the question of induction is mooted.

Suggestions that women in some other centres regard oxytocin with suspicion and, in the event of slow progress, frequently decline acceleration, could only be the result of misunderstandings which, in turn, reflect poorly on the quality of the educational service. Paradoxically, induction rates, which involve identical procedures, may be high in these same centres. The authors never cease to be impressed by the ability of the average woman to assimilate the essential facts about labour when these are properly presented.

Key Points

- Expectant mothers should be made aware that childbirth is primarily their responsibility
- Adequate educational servives should be readily available to all expectant mothers, particularly nulliparous women

Care of Fetus   **23**

Overall care of the fetus during labour is based on the simple premise that the fetus who presents as a case of hypoxia during the course of normal labour is almost sure to have been compromised before labour began. The occasional exception is likely to be the result of an accident of labour, which causes acute hypoxia in a hitherto normal fetus: prolapse of cord is the classic example. The aims, therefore, are two-fold: first, to identify the fetus who is already affected and, second, to ensure that the labour itself remains normal.[12]

Artificial rupture of membranes

To identify the fetus who may already be compromised, artificial rupture of membranes is performed as soon as a formal diagnosis of labour is made and the woman is, therefore, committed to delivery. A free flow of clear liquor is regarded as strong evidence that the function of the placenta should be sufficient to withstand the pressures of normal labour. A sample of liquor is retained in a test tube for inspection in every case.

This procedure is intended to identify cases that have escaped detection in late pregnancy, before the additional stress of labour can cause an already precarious balance to deteriorate abruptly.

Meconium

Meconium is regarded as a clinical sign of great potential significance. At the outset, women in labour are divided into two groups: those with clear liquor and those with meconium. The division into low-risk and high-risk cases is made on this simple evidence which is of direct fetal origin.

Not all meconium, however, is accorded the same significance. There is a world of difference between light meconium staining of a large volume of liquor and meconium that is virtually undiluted, with umbilical cord, membranes and even endometrium coloured green through its entire depth when exposed subsequently at caesarean section.

Meconium is interpreted as evidence of placental insufficiency of some duration, not as evidence of short-term fetal distress. Moreover, meconium seldom appears for the first time during the course of normal labour.

Three grades of meconium are recognized, as follows:

Grade I   A good volume of liquor stained lightly with meconium.
Grade II   A reasonable volume of liquor with a heavy suspension of meconium.
Grade III   Thick meconium which is undiluted with liquor and resembles
              sieved spinach.

All grades of meconium are reported to the senior registrar. Continuous cardio-tocography is commenced in all cases. A wide margin of discretion is permitted in Grade I; after careful review of all the clinical circumstances no further action is taken in most cases. In Grade II; treatment is determined by the fetal heart rate pattern. Caesarean section is performed in Grade III unless an easy vaginal delivery is imminent; not only hypoxia but also meconium inhalation is a real possibility in this situation.

No liquor

Failure to recover any liquor at artificial rupture of membranes is, for reasons of safety, treated as meconium Grade II, although clear liquor frequently appears at a later stage.

Fetal heart

Direct auscultation of the fetal heart is a duty performed by the personal midwife who supervises each labour. This is for one full minute, at intervals of 15 minutes during the first stage, and after each contraction during the second stage.

Routine electronic monitoring is not practised in the National Maternity Hospital; it is used for specific indications only. Routine electronic monitoring of the fetal heart during labour affords no additional protection against cerebral palsy[13,14] and electronic monitors, without fetal blood sampling as a control, lead to a sharp increase in the caesarean section rate for suspected fetal distress.

Fetal blood sample

Fetal acidosis is accepted as the definitive test for hypoxia. Only in exceptional circumstances is a woman subjected to caesarean section for the indication fetal distress without this confirmation. In practice, this situation is likely to arise most frequently in the presence of Grade II meconium, where caesarean section would have to be performed – sometimes unnecessarily – were the definitive test not available.

Normal labour

Since the contention is that normal placental function is sufficient to sustain the fetus through the exigencies of normal labour, it is necessary to have a clear understanding of what is meant by this term. Labour is defined as normal when delivery is effected within 12 hours through the efforts of the mother, although this need not preclude use of simple vaginal operative delivery in this instance. Steps taken to ensure that labour conforms to this definition of normality would appear to be a valuable contribution to the welfare of the fetus. Trauma is to be avoided at all costs, and trauma is least likely to occur when mothers deliver themselves.

Key Points

- The fetus who enters labour in good condition is equipped by nature to withstand the challenge of normal birth

- Electronic fetal monitoring is for specifically indicated purposes only

- Routine electronic monitoring does not reduce the incidence of cereral palsy

- Ideally fetal blood sampling should be used to confirm fetal distress before caesarean section is undertaken

Induction   **24**

This manual is not concerned with induction as a separate entity but only in-directly, in so far as it may impinge on the conduct of labour. The relationship was discussed briefly in Chapter 2, where two points were emphasized: first, that there should be no confusion between induction and acceleration and, second, that induction has a profound effect on the care of labour as a whole. Furthermore, the adverse effects of induction are by no means confined to the individuals directly involved: they extend to everyone delivered in a hospital in which induction is freely practised. Against this background, there are three different aspects of induction which merit close attention: indications, suitability and methods.[15]

Indications

The laxity, or otherwise, of the indications for induction best illustrates the magni-tude of the iatrogenic problem created by this form of medical intervention, in each institution. One of many unfortunate consequences of an uncritical applica-tion of audit to obstetric practice in recent years has been an increase in undefined indications for induction of labour. Pre-eclampsia and prolonged pregnancy are the two outstanding examples; these are the indications recorded in a large majority of cases, whether the incidence of the procedure be high or low. Although perinatal and maternal morbidity and mortality may increase in these conditions, the adverse effect of an increased induction rate must not be underestimated. The result is that a high proportion of cases on whom induction is performed for pre-eclampsia or prolonged pregnancy – or other equally undefined category – do not conform to any critical assessment. Furthermore, even in the minority of cases who do conform to critical assessment, the likelihood of an unfavourable outcome is so small that it does not justify a routine approach, where many are subjected to a potentially hazardous form of treatment in the hope that a few might benefit. So-called 'induction of labour' is undertaken far too often on a rule-of-thumb basis with little attempt to select the individuals who are genuinely in need of delivery.

Suitability

The standard of suitability adopted largely determines the number of failures. As the indication for delivery is seldom absolute, the decision to proceed with induction should be subject to the likelihood of success in each instance.

Induction is best attempted when the head is engaged and the cervix is favourable. Whenever the need to interrupt the course of pregnancy arises before these basic conditions are fulfilled, caesarean section may be performed on the grounds that induction is not the correct method of treatment in these circumstances.

An implication that the end justifies the means in this context, and that whatever transpires subsequently can be blamed on the condition for which the induction was nominally performed, is not tenable. In all walks of life prudence requires that no action be taken without due consideration of possible consequences; this is certainly true of obstetrics. The decision to interrupt the course of pregnancy is a clear example of a balance of risks. Selecting induction as the method of achieving this end may be correct in one instance, where conditions are favourable, but incorrect in another, where conditions are unfavourable. Far too many inductions are undertaken for dubious reasons in unfavourable circumstances, with the result that the treatment is more dangerous than the indication given for induction. An uncritical approach to this potentially serious issue is the cause of considerable disquiet, which is not confined to obstetricians.

Method

The method of induction determines the length of time spent in a delivery unit by women who are not yet in labour. This consideration has important consequences, both for those individuals directly involved, and for all other women who share the facilities of a delivery unit where there are a large number of inductions. To reduce time spent in the delivery unit by women not yet in labour – primarily for their own comfort, but also in the general interest – the method of induction favoured in the National Maternity Hospital consists of simple amniotomy. The final decision to proceed with amniotomy is taken at pelvic examination by a doctor with the status of senior registrar. The membranes are ruptured at a fixed time of day, and the woman remains in the antenatal ward to await the onset of labour. Meanwhile, no restrictions are placed on her movements. The result is that 90% of women subjected to amniotomy for the purpose of induction are already in labour when they enter the delivery unit. Subsequent progress is similar in all respects to that of women admitted from their homes, whether this is expressed in terms of hours spent in the delivery unit, drugs administered for relief of pain or operative procedures undertaken. Prostaglandin is used to ripen the cervix prior to amniotomy in selected cases.

Labour does not begin within 24 hours of amniotomy in 10% of cases; these are officially recorded as failed inductions. Next morning, these 'failed inductions' – so classified because they did not respond to simple amniotomy – are transferred to the delivery unit where oxytocin is given as a back-up procedure. The same solution and rate as for acceleration of labour is used: 10 units in 1 litre of normal saline. The result is that 90% of these exceptional cases deliver vaginally within 12 hours. Caesarean section is performed when labour is not well advanced after 1 litre – which requires 6 hours – or, in any event, after a woman has been in the delivery unit for 12 hours.

This method of procedure ensures that few women admitted to the delivery unit receive oxytocin for the purpose of induction. The contribution made by this simple arrangement to the overall quality of care afforded to the totality of women in labour is enormous. Facilities, especially in terms of human resources, are not dissipated in the care of women who are not in labour and who, therefore, should not be in a delivery unit. There are many delivery units in which – at any given time – one in every two women is not in labour. Nonetheless, these are the women who attract most attention, and for a much longer time. This attention can only be made available at the expense of the women who are in labour.

The main argument advanced in support of the immediate use of oxytocin, after amniotomy, to induce labour is based on the fact that the likelihood of infection increases with the passage of time: the induction–delivery interval. In practice, however, the risk is small when cases are carefully selected and delivery is almost sure to take place within 24 hours. Under these circumstances, the risk of infection is certainly not sufficient to justify serious disruption of an entire service by the admission of a large number of women who are not in labour. This is a good example of the balance of risks applied to a much wider issue.

Key Points

- There are direct and indirect adverse effects of a high induction rate
- Induction of labour should be restricted to a select number of individuals in which the indication is genuine and conditions are favourable
- Critical audit of indications and outcome of induction is mandatory
- The methods of induction should be chosen to cause least disturbance to the individual and least disruption to the service

Organization   25

Although there may be other fields of clinical practice of which it could be said with equal truth that more is to be gained from sound organizational methods than from sophisticated techniques, there can be few more obvious examples than a modern delivery unit. No matter how sophisticated the equipment may become, a delivery unit cannot begin to function properly unless the basic organization is sound.[16]

Delivery units, in general, suffer from poor organizational standards, mainly because they lack central direction; in terms of care they often border on the chaotic – unable to cope with occasional additional pressures even though overstaffed for much of the time. Corporate spirit tends to be poorly developed, with midwives, doctors and even administrators failing to cooperate closely with each other, even within the same group. Sometimes they may actually be in open conflict. Inevitably, wherever this situation exists, it operates to the detriment of the patients.

Better organization can transform the quality of care afforded to women in labour; in addition, it can greatly enhance the level of job satisfaction of professional staff and provide an objective basis for costs incurred in a very expensive service. As is so often the case, good practice corresponds with good economics in this instance. Both make good sense.

Midwifery services

In terms of organization, the key to the solution of the problems of a modern delivery unit lies in the midwifery service. Midwifery staff must be deployed for the declared purpose of providing professional attention at personal level for every woman in labour. The same number of midwives, of equal status, must operate day and night, as concrete evidence of the fact that the welfare of mothers and infants is not to be influenced by the time at which a birth happens to occur. This cannot be achieved through a haphazard approach: careful planning is needed.

Scale

A large-scale operation confers an obvious advantage in this respect because it helps to eliminate peaks and troughs in terms of numbers of babies born at different hours of the day, days of the week or seasons of the year. In the National

Maternity Hospital, currently with some 8000 deliveries per annum, the percentage of total births which occur in each of the 8-hour periods corresponding with official working shifts falls between 30 and 35 and, in each month, between 7.5 and 9.5. This provides a reasonably even distribution at all times. Furthermore, scale permits a nucleus of highly skilled midwives to be employed on a whole-time commitment to the delivery unit, so that they are not required to divide their attention with antenatal or postnatal wards, nor to leave women in labour to assist at caesarean sections.

Intensive care

Nowadays, delivery units are frequently spoken of in the context of intensive care, although services, especially midwifery services, continue to function in a largely fragmentary manner, devoid of any rational explanation and heavily concentrated in daylight hours. This arrangement, it would appear, is to suit staff rather than 'patients'. There is a wide credibility gap here that needs to be closed.

Bottleneck

In every maternity unit the delivery unit represents a bottleneck through which all mothers must pass. Hence, it is here that the number of confinements for which the entire system can cater is determined. Accommodation elsewhere, especially in postnatal wards that comprise the bulk of obstetrical beds, is extremely flexible. The immediate effect of a general reduction of stay in a postnatal ward by one day would be to increase the functional capacity of a maternity unit by at least 20%. These are considerations of great practical importance in terms of public expenditure at current levels. In a maternity service, only a special care baby unit can compare with a labour ward in terms of concentration of expertise, with corresponding costs. Both should be efficiently used. Antenatal and postnatal wards are areas of comparatively low-level care where most mothers can, and indeed should, fend largely for themselves.

Duration of stay

The ability to limit the duration of labour and, therefore, calculate the total number of hours to be serviced, has transformed the previously haphazard approach to planning in this department. To take a simple example: one midwife in the course of her working day can supervise one woman during a labour which lasts 8 hours, whereas three midwives are required to supervise the same woman during a labour which lasts 24 hours. The problem is compounded by extensive use of induction, where midwives are engaged in looking after women who, for much of the time, are not in labour. A liberal attitude towards induction constitutes an almost insurmountable barrier to the application of sound organizational methods in a delivery unit, especially where the central issue of midwifery services is concerned.

The practice

There were 7840 babies born in the National Maternity Hospital during the year 2000. The total midwifery complement employed whole-time in the delivery unit was 53 (33 graduate and 20 student midwives). This complement includes provision for holiday relief and other off-duty situations such as study leave and occasional illness. There was no other category of nursing attendant involved. Hence, the average number of babies born for each midwife employed was 148. This compares with a corresponding number of 207 in 1970, when 6225 babies were born. The latter figure was the subject of a report in *Proceedings of the Royal Society of Medicine*, where comparison was made with an average figure of 84 births for each midwife employed in the delivery unit, in a sample of five similar institutions around the British Isles. The unit cost of production, relating salaries paid to midwives to number of babies born, was three times higher in the other five centres, although the level of remuneration was comparable. Paradoxically, this was the only one of the six units surveyed where a personal midwife was provided for every woman in labour.

Each midwifery team on duty in the National Maternity Hospital consists of one Sister, four staff midwives and four student midwives. In addition, there is one medical student who performs the same duties as the student midwife.

To ensure that every woman in labour has continuous personal attention one student is allotted to each room. Staff midwives act mainly in a supervisory capacity, with the Sister in complete overall control. Hence the unit cost of production, in which midwives' salaries are by far the largest item, can be readily estimated. This provides a basis of comparison from year to year and between one institution and another.

Although none is nearly as important as the midwifery element, there are other aspects of the comprehensive organizational requirement of an efficient delivery service which, hopefully, may have been discerned as a continuous thread running through the pages of this text. Most important is the need for central direction to draw the diverse elements together, thus welding a team out of a collection of individuals of various disciplines and different levels of seniority. The result should be an efficient, happy and economical unit which is seen to make sense to all who work there.

Key Points

- Duration of labour is associated with the ability to combine a nucleus of skilled midwives with personal attention for every woman in labour
- Good organization contributes more to care in labour than any number of sophisticated techniques

Cervix in Labour   26

Obstetrics suffers grievously from lack of accurate definition, not only of common clinical conditions – of which labour itself is a prime example – but also of terms commonly used to describe essential features of these conditions. One suspects that if several individuals who worked in the same delivery unit, and who had long grown accustomed to exchange these mundane terms on a daily basis, were asked what precisely they understood the words 'effacement' and 'dilatation' to mean or, better still, were presented with pencil and paper and asked to reproduce them as simple line drawings, the results would be very different. Yet few would dispute that it is a matter of considerable practical consequence that there should be, at the very least, a common language amongst workers in the same medical field.

Parity factor

In preceding chapters, attention has repeatedly been drawn to the need to consider nulliparous and parous women completely differently in all matters relating to labour. The cervix is one more example. To the examining finger, the nulliparous cervix and the parous cervix are so widely dissimilar that they could well be different organs. The greatest difference concerns the external os which remains permanently ajar after the birth of a first child. Herein lies a source of endless confusion; hence, the parity factor must be taken into account whenever the terms 'effacement' and 'dilatation' are under consideration. The best way to illustrate this statement is by diagrammatic representation (see *Figure 26.1*).

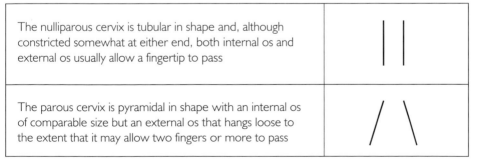

The nulliparous cervix is tubular in shape and, although constricted somewhat at either end, both internal os and external os usually allow a fingertip to pass	
The parous cervix is pyramidal in shape with an internal os of comparable size but an external os that hangs loose to the extent that it may allow two fingers or more to pass	

Figure 26.1 Diagrammatic representation of the nulliparous and the parous cervix.

Effacement

Effacement is the process of inclusion of the entire length of cervical canal into the lower segment, or body, of uterus. This begins at the internal os and proceeds downwards to the external os, at which level effacement is complete (see *Figure 26.2*). The process of effacement may occur late in pregnancy or be delayed in its entirety until labour begins. An important corollary is that effacement of cervix is not an essential requirement for a diagnosis of labour: a woman may be in labour without her cervix being effaced, much less dilated, thus emphasizing the practical importance of a 'show' or spontaneous rupture of membranes, as discussed in

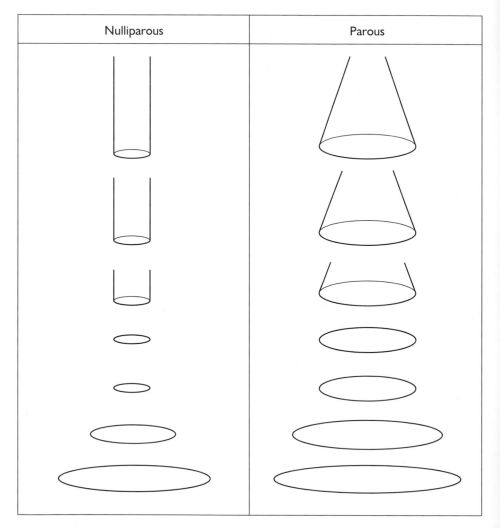

Nulliparous	Parous

Figure 26.2 Diagrammatic representation of process of effacement followed by dilatation of the nulliparous and the parous cervix.

Chapter 5. However, in the event of effacement not having taken place to some extent beforehand, duration of labour is likely to be prolonged. These are usually the troublesome cases.

Dilatation

Dilatation refers to the external os only. The external os cannot begin to open until the process of effacement is complete. Effacement and dilatation are consecutive, not simultaneous, events. This sequential relationship is of paramount importance: a cervix which is not effaced cannot possibly be dilated, even though, as is often the case in a parous woman, the external os may freely admit two fingers at pelvic examination. The patulous state of the external os in a parous woman is a relic of a previous birth; it is passive in nature and must not be confused with the active process of dilatation which denotes labour here and now. Naturally, therefore, by the time a parous cervix achieves full effacement it is already the equivalent of 2 cm open on the dilatation scale.

Transition

The point of transition, where effacement ends and dilatation begins, requires special attention. At this point the presence or absence of painful uterine contractions is decisive. Since without painful uterine contractions there is no question of a woman being in labour, a fully effaced cervix in these circumstances should be said to admit one or more fingers, as the case may be, whereas with painful uterine contractions the same cervix should be said to be dilated to the extent of 1 cm or more. The former expression is intended to convey an inert or static situation, the latter to convey an evolving or dynamic situation.

Key Points

- It should be recognized that many of the problems encountered in a delivery unit have their origin in an inability to diagnose labour correctly
- Surprisingly little attention is directed to the meaning of the terms used to describe the sequence of events at this crucial time

Caesarean Section Rates   27

Background

The most significant development in childbirth over the past 35 years has been the increase in the number of deliveries by caesarean section that has taken place to a greater or lesser extent worldwide. This increase can only be justified by improved perinatal or maternal outcome. There is, however, a dearth of detailed, consistent, standardized information being collected by delivery units on outcome. This does not allow the continuous critical review which is the foundation of the philosophy of Active Management of Labour. The problem with interpreting any available evidence is the lack of consistency of definitions and classification. Furthermore, cause and effect need to be determined if progress is to be made. It is a matter of the utmost importance that facile conclusions in respect of cause and effect relationships between caesarean section rates and perinatal mortality and morbidity outcome as well as maternal outcome are continuously challenged.

Counting the cost

Given the lack of evidence that the massive increase in caesarean rates throughout much of the western world has resulted in any tangible benefits for infants, there are some pertinent questions to be asked:

- Does it really matter what the caesarean section rate is in a particular hospital or community?
- At individual level, is it a matter of any great consequence that a woman's first baby is delivered by caesarean section, possibly under epidural anaesthesia with her husband present, if she is not likely to have more than two children in any event?
- For the obstetrician, who carries a dual responsibility, are there considerations of professional ethics in so far as the mother's welfare is concerned?
- Who created the medicolegal climate which is said to be a factor in many countries, and dominant in some?
- Finally, and perhaps most important of all, what are the repercussions of this radical change in practice on the Third World, many of whose graduates are trained in western methods?

Sooner or later these questions will have to be answered; they cannot be avoided indefinitely, as caesarean section rates continue to rise.

Classification of caesarean sections

Much has been written about caesarean section rates and their associated factors. However, these rates have not been classified in a way that would allow consistent interpretation and identify areas where care could be assessed more closely and improved. Any classification also needs to be linked to perinatal and maternal outcome so that their relationships can be studied.

The caesarean section rate in the National Maternity Hospital increased from 5.1% in 1985 to 14.2% in 2000. Since 1992 caesarean sections have been classified using a new system[17] which helps interpret changes in caesarean section rates. The system is based on looking at caesarean section rates in different groups of women according to the following obstetric concepts:

- whether the woman is nulliparous, multiparous without a scar or multiparous with a scar
- whether the pregnancy is single cephalic, single breech, a multiple pregnancy, or a transverse or oblique lie
- whether labour is spontaneous or induced, or delivery took place by caesarean section before labour
- the gestational age of the pregnancy.

Ten groups of women are identified: all prospective, mutually exclusive, totally inclusive, easily identifiable and clinically relevant. The 10 groups are intended to give an overview of a caesarean section rate which thus can be easily compared. After the initial comparison, individual groups are identified which can be examined in more detail to determine the reasons for differences. Indications for caesarean section are only useful after the classification into the different groups, as definitions of indications will vary between the groups, as will the management of the groups.

Reasons for the increase

The National Institutes of Health Consensus Development Report on Cesarean Childbirth[18] clearly identified dystocia, or abnormal labour, as the main reason for the rapid expansion of caesarean section in the USA: more specifically, dystocia in nulliparous women with a single cephalic pregnancy in labour, which is the central issue of this book. Parous women do not suffer from dystocia to any significant extent. The most important consequence of this is that the more primary caesarean sections performed today, the more secondary caesarean sections will be necessary tomorrow.

Although the caesarean section rate has increased in the National Maternity Hospital since 1985, the incidence in nulliparous women with a single cephalic pregnancy in spontaneous labour has remained constant. The low caesarean section rate for dystocia in this group of women which has continued at the National Maternity Hospital through the intervening years must be seen as testimony to the fundamental truth: that efficient uterine action is the key to normal labour.

The rise in the number of caesarean sections carried out for other reasons must not be allowed to go unchallenged. As with induction of labour, the lack of definition of the indications for caesarean section increases the magnitude of the iatrogenic problem created. One of many unfortunate consequences of an uncritical application of audit to obstetric practice in recent years has been an increase in undefined indications for induction of labour and caesarean section.

Key Points

- There has been a worldwide increase in caesarean section rates in recent years
- A standard classification of caesarean section rates is required
- Most of the increase has been in spontaneously labouring, nulliparous women with a single cephalic pregnancy for the indication dystocia
- The problem of dystocia can be solved by ensuring efficient uterine action
- The more primary caesarean sections performed today, the more secondary caesarean sections will be necessary tomorrow

Cerebral Palsy   28

The influence of perinatal factors on subsequent neurological development is a dominant concern in the wider context of reproductive medicine. Brain damage that could have been avoided may well be regarded as the ultimate failure in contemporary obstetric care. The traditional viewpoint – entrenched in the minds of many obstetricians, paediatricians and, indeed, the community at large – that cerebral palsy is almost invariably the result of asphyxia during labour, is seriously challenged by the results of the Dublin Trial, so called because it was conducted in the National Maternity Hospital.[13,19]

Hypoxia

Labour is a potential cause of asphyxia because blood flow through the placenta is always impeded by uterine activity: every uterine contraction reduces oxygen supply to the fetus. As labour progresses, the cumulative effect may lead to a significant degree of hypoxia. This physiological process presents no problem to the well-nourished fetus who enters labour with a normal placenta and sufficient reserve to adapt to labour of reasonable duration. On the other hand, the fetus whose reserve is already diminished before labour begins is vulnerable to the stress of normal labour. To the fetus, the consequence is the same whether the natural action of the uterus is sufficient to dilate the cervix or inefficient uterine action is corrected with oxytocin.

Care of fetus during labour

Supervision of the fetus during labour is based on the simple premise that a healthy fetus and placenta are generally competent to meet the stress of normal labour. To ensure early detection of a fetus who is already compromised by impaired placental function, but which has escaped recognition at the antenatal clinic, amniotomy is performed as soon as the diagnosis of labour is confirmed. Given clear liquor, supervision thereafter is by intermittent auscultation, performed for one full minute, at intervals of 15 minutes during the first stage and after every contraction during the second stage, unless specific signs indicate the need for electronic fetal monitoring and possible fetal blood sampling.

Research project

Because of the long-running controversy concerning the respective values of continuous electronic monitoring and intermittent auscultation, a decision was made to compare the two methods in the context of the practice of the National Maternity Hospital. Certain cases were specifically excluded from the trial beforehand, i.e. those with meconium or no liquor at rupture of membranes; these represented 6% of the total. All other cases were included, without regard to risk status by conventional standards such as pre-eclampsia, antepartum haemorrhage or diabetes. The number of eligible cases was 12 964, of which 6474 were allocated on a random basis to the continuous electronically monitored group and 6490 to the intermittently auscultated group. Both groups used fetal blood sampling to confirm fetal distress.

The results showed no difference in perinatal mortality rates – 14 deaths in each group. Neither was there a significant difference in Apgar scores, need for intubation, or admission to the Special Care Baby Unit. There was one significant difference: the incidence of neonatal convulsions in those who survived. There were nine cases of neonatal convulsions in the electronically monitored group, compared with 21 in the intermittently auscultated group. When these 30 infants were examined after 12 months, six showed evidence of permanent damage, all of the cerebral palsy type: three were from the electronically monitored group and three were from the intermittently auscultated group.[13,14]

Significantly, the perinatal mortality rate in cases excluded from the trial on the basis of meconium or no liquor was five times greater than the overall figure for cases included. The caesarean section rate was low and not significantly different in either of the study groups: 2.4% and 2.2%, respectively. Elective caesarean sections are, of course, not represented here. The close similarity between the two groups is almost certainly the result of retaining the blood sample as the final arbiter of distress in both instances. There can be little doubt that electronic monitoring, without the benefit of fetal blood sampling, leads to a sharp increase in the caesarean section rate for the indication fetal distress with no apparent benefit.

At 4 years of age, reassessment of the 30 children who had survived neonatal convulsions confirmed that six suffered from cerebral palsy: the same three from each group. A fourth child from the electronic group found to have cerebral palsy at 4 years had had transient neurological signs during the neonatal period. There were, in addition, 15 other cases of cerebral palsy who had had no abnormal signs during the neonatal period: eight from the electronic group and seven from the intermittently auscultated group. At the end of 4 years, therefore, there were 22 cases of cerebral palsy: 12 from the electronic group and 10 from the intermittently auscultated group. A finding of at least equal importance to the practice of obstetrics was that only six of the 22 cases of cerebral palsy at 4 years of age had shown any sign of hypoxia at birth.

Two firm conclusions are drawn from this study: first, that routine continuous electronic monitoring of the fetal heart during labour afforded no additional protection against cerebral palsy and, second, that cerebral palsy was not associated with hypoxia at birth in most cases.

Key Points

- Routine use of electronic monitoring in labour does not reduce the incidence of cerebral palsy
- Most cases of cerebral palsy are not associated with hypoxia in labour

Section II
Visual Records of Labour

Nulliparous Labour

Nulliparous labour

There are fundamental differences between first and all subsequent labours. These differences are so great that they warrant the statement that nulliparous and parous women behave as different biological species; proper care of labour rests on this basic premise.

- The causes of delay and risks of treatment are very different.
- The duration of a first labour is longer because inefficient uterine action is commonplace and because the birth canal has not been stretched before.
- Inefficient uterine action is uncommon in parous women. Delay in parous labour is often an expression of obstruction caused by a fetal complication, such as malformation or malpresentation, which can easily lead to rupture of uterus.
- The nulliparous uterus is immune to rupture.
- The parous uterus is prone to rupture.
- Oxytocin does not cause rupture of the nulliparous uterus, even in the presence of cephalopelvic disproportion.
- Oxytocin may cause rupture of the parous uterus in normal labour.
- To ensure that this distinction is manifest at all times the Nulliparous Labour Record is printed on yellow paper and the Parous Labour Record on blue paper.

PARTOGRAM 1

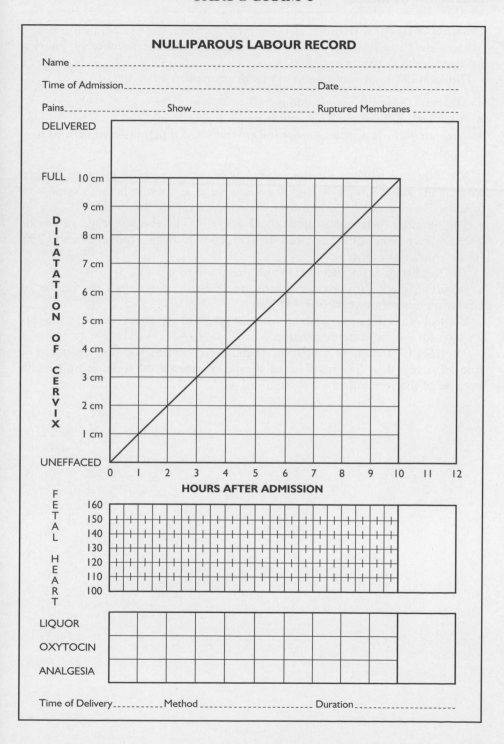

NULLIPAROUS LABOUR RECORD

Name _____

Time of Admission _____ Date _____

Pains _____ Show _____ Ruptured Membranes _____

DELIVERED

FULL   10 cm
         9 cm
D   8 cm
I
L   7 cm
A
T   6 cm
A
T   5 cm
I
O   4 cm
N
         3 cm
O
F   2 cm

C   1 cm
E
R
V
I
X
UNEFFACED

DILATATION OF CERVIX

0   1   2   3   4   5   6   7   8   9   10   11   12

HOURS AFTER ADMISSION

F   160
E   150
T   140
A
L   130
         120
H   110
E   100
A
R
T

FETAL HEART

LIQUOR

OXYTOCIN

ANALGESIA

Time of Delivery _____ Method _____ Duration _____

Duration of labour

Duration of labour is recorded as the interval between time of admission to the delivery unit and time of delivery. This equates with the number of hours a woman spends in the delivery unit.

Duration of labour is expressed in this manner because:

- Mothers decide the time of admission.
- Attendant staff assume their responsibility at this point.
- Accurate records demand precise information which permits comparisons to be made.

No allowance is made for time spent at home. It is self-evident that every woman in whom labour is confirmed has been in labour before coming to hospital. To estimate duration from such evidence is pure guesswork.

The duration of labour is determined effectively by the first stage of labour because the number of hours taken for the cervix to dilate represents some 90% of the entire birth process.

The third stage is not included in this definition of labour.

Duration, more than any other measurable factor, determines the impact of labour on mothers in particular, but also on babies.

Control of the duration of labour without resort to caesarean section represents a major advance in obstetric practice.

The mean duration of labour in nulliparous women without treatment is somewhat less than 6 hours. Use of the term 'average duration' is misleading because of the very wide natural variation.

PARTOGRAM 2

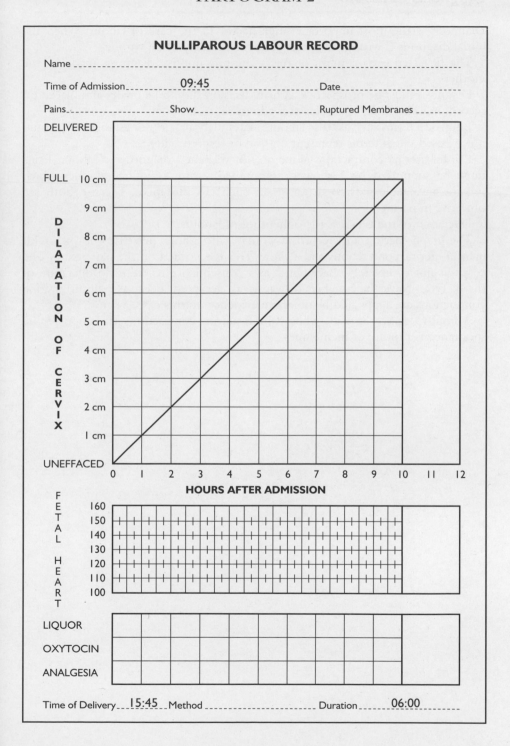

Diagnosis of labour

Diagnosis is the most important single factor in the care of labour. When the initial diagnosis is wrong, all subsequent care is likely to be wrong.

The first step is to confirm or reject the presumptive diagnosis made by the mother.

Diagnosis must be prospective. A firm decision should be made, and placed on record, not later than one hour after admission to hospital.

Equivocal terms such as 'false labour', 'latent labour' or 'not established' should not be used. Such terms represent evasion of responsibility.

Painful uterine contractions alone do not warrant a diagnosis of labour. Pains must be supported by a show or spontaneous rupture of membranes which provide invaluable aids to diagnosis in such circumstances, because both are objective in nature.

Dilatation of the cervix is the only proof of labour.

The graph (partogram) records a woman who admits herself to hospital with painful uterine contractions and a show. This is recorded on the partogram. The cervix is not completely effaced and, as a consequence, there is no dilatation of the cervix. Nevertheless, her diagnosis is accepted because painful uterine contractions are supported by objective evidence: in this case, a show.

A similar decision is made when painful uterine contractions are supported by spontaneous rupture of membranes.

PARTOGRAM 3

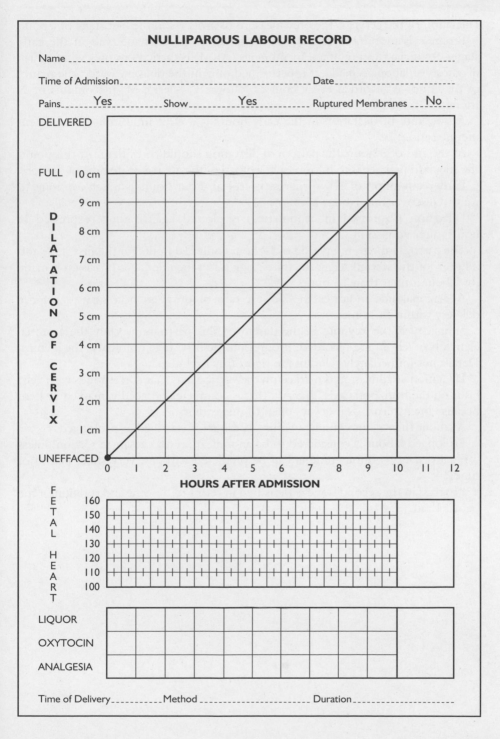

NULLIPAROUS LABOUR RECORD

Name _____

Time of Admission _____ Date _____

Pains _____ Yes _____ Show _____ Yes _____ Ruptured Membranes ___ No ___

Progress in labour

Dilatation of the cervix is the only measure of progress in the first stage of labour.

Progress is monitored by vaginal examination at short intervals in the early stages. Artificial rupture of the membranes (ARM) is carried out only when a firm diagnosis of labour is made; it is performed only in the delivery ward. The nature of the liquor is recorded every hour as follows: C (clear), M (meconium) or N (none).

A slow rate of dilatation in the early hours is a clear indication of inefficient uterine action.

At the end of 3 hours the pattern of dilatation should be evident. At this point, the standard practice is to inform each woman of the approximate time of delivery.

Early recognition of slow progress is crucial. Four hours is much too long to wait to discover that labour is abnormal.

Dilatation (expressed in centimetres) is plotted against time (expressed in hours) after admission.

The partogram covers a period of 12 hours only: 10 hours for the first stage and 2 hours for the second stage; the third stage is not included. No provision is made for labour longer than 12 hours.

A diagonal line indicates the slowest rate of progress necessary to achieve delivery within this time.

Simplicity is the keynote in the design of this partogram. Only the essential elements of labour are recorded. Progress in the first stage dominates the picture. Details not immediately relevant are rigorously excluded.

Dilatation at admission is marked on the vertical axis that corresponds with zero hour on the horizontal axis. A cervix that is completely effaced is marked at 1 cm because the external os is always open to this extent.

A labour that is not complete within 12 hours is classified as prolonged.

Prolonged labour is considered to be an indication for caesarean section unless vaginal delivery without trauma can be predicted within a very short period of time.

Progress in the second stage is measured in terms of descent and rotation of the baby's head.

PARTOGRAM 4

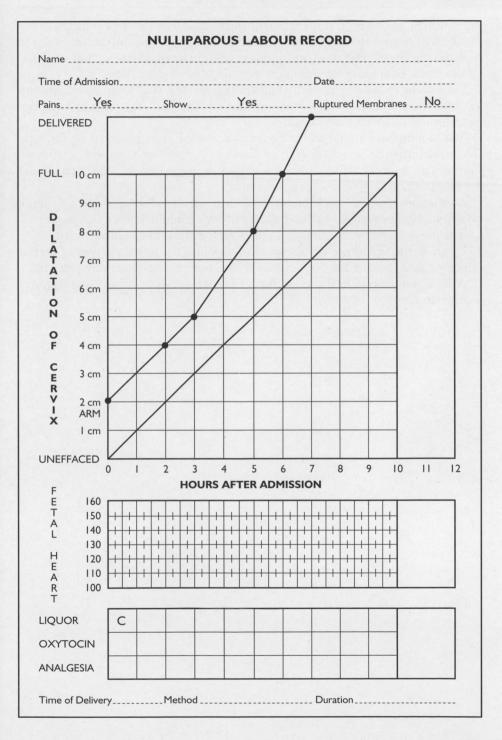

NULLIPAROUS LABOUR RECORD

Name _____

Time of Admission _____ Date _____

Pains _____ Yes _____ Show _____ Yes _____ Ruptured Membranes ___ No ___

DELIVERED

FULL

DILATATION OF CERVIX

10 cm
9 cm
8 cm
7 cm
6 cm
5 cm
4 cm
3 cm
2 cm ARM
1 cm

UNEFFACED

0 1 2 3 4 5 6 7 8 9 10 11 12

HOURS AFTER ADMISSION

FETAL HEART

160
150
140
130
120
110
100

LIQUOR   C

OXYTOCIN

ANALGESIA

Time of Delivery _____ Method _____ Duration _____

Care of the fetus

Intermittent auscultation is the standard method of fetal heart monitoring.

The fetal heart is recorded by the personal midwife for one full minute every 15 minutes during the first stage and after every contraction in the second stage.

Electronic fetal heart monitoring is used in selected cases only.

Fetal scalp blood pH is the definitive test for hypoxia. Only in exceptional circumstances is caesarean section performed for fetal distress without prior examination of a fetal scalp sample.

The amount and colour of the liquor is accorded great potential significance. To enable inspection of the liquor, amniotomy is performed as soon as labour is confirmed. A good volume of clear liquor is regarded as almost conclusive evidence of normal feto-placental function.

Meconium raises a suspicion of fetal hypoxia, as does absence of liquor. Attention is drawn to the different grades of meconium described in Chapter 23.

The use of oxytocin is prohibited unless fetal distress has been excluded.

Grade II meconium, or no liquor, is an absolute bar to stimulation of uterine activity unless hypoxia has been excluded by a normal fetal heart rate pattern.

A high standard of fetal monitoring in labour does not require sophisticated equipment.

PARTOGRAM 5

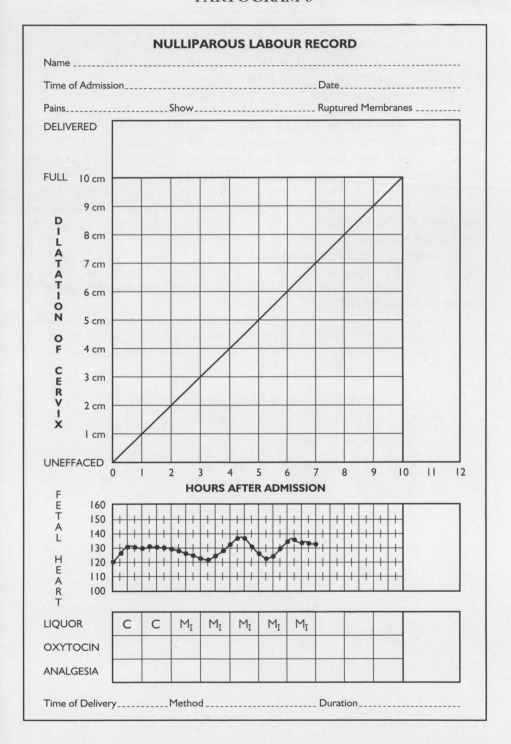

NULLIPAROUS LABOUR RECORD

Name _____

Time of Admission _____ Date _____

Pains _____ Show _____ Ruptured Membranes _____

DELIVERED

FULL 10 cm
9 cm
8 cm
7 cm
6 cm
5 cm
4 cm
3 cm
2 cm
1 cm
UNEFFACED

D I L A T A T I O N   O F   C E R V I X

0   1   2   3   4   5   6   7   8   9   10   11   12

HOURS AFTER ADMISSION

F E T A L   H E A R T
160
150
140
130
120
110
100

LIQUOR	C	C	M$_I$	M$_I$	M$_I$	M$_I$	M$_I$			
OXYTOCIN										
ANALGESIA										

Time of Delivery _____ Method _____ Duration _____

Oxytocin

Oxytocin (indicated in red on the partogram) provides a safe and simple treatment of slow labour in the nulliparous woman, provided rigid rules are enforced.

A standard concentration of 10 units in 1 litre of normal saline is used. In no circumstance is this concentration changed.

The total dose of oxytocin may not exceed 10 units.

The rate of infusion begins at 10 drops and increases by 10 drops every 15 minutes to a maximum of 60 drops per minute (40 milliunits/minute). The concentration, the rate and the volume must not be exceeded.

The infusion may be administered by a simple gravity feed which is regulated by the personal midwife.

The number of contractions during each period of 15 minutes is recorded in serial fashion on the reverse side of the chart. The aim is five contractions in each period of 15 minutes. Should the frequency of contractions exceed seven, the infusion rate is reduced to guard against hypertonus.

Intrauterine pressures are not recorded.

Oxytocin is an extraordinarily effective drug when used to accelerate labour, but its effectiveness is often inhibited by fear of cephalopelvic disproportion, rupture of the uterus and trauma to the baby.

A fundamental distinction must be made between nulliparous and parous women. Oxytocin should only be used with utmost caution in parous women.

Management of dystocia in nulliparous women demands the use of oxytocin.

Time	Rate	Contractions
12.00	10	1,2
12.15	20	3,4,5
12.30	30	6,7,8
12.45	40	9,10,11
13.00	50	12,13,14,15
13.15	60	16,17,18,19,20

PARTOGRAM 6

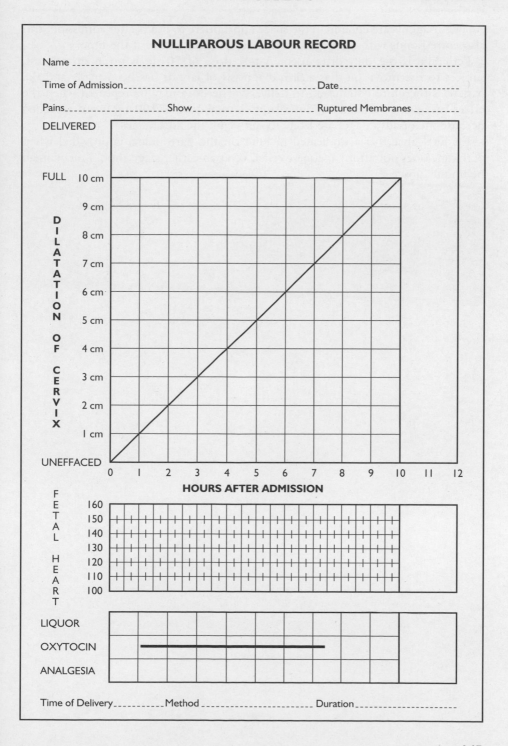

Analgesia

Analgesic agents are entered in the space appropriate to hours after admission; this also corresponds with the degree of dilatation of the cervix at the time.

Pethidine is the only drug used. A test dose of 50 mg is given on request, subject to the provision that a firm diagnosis of labour has been made and the patient is therefore committed to delivery. The dose may be repeated when the effect has been assessed 30 minutes later. A total dose of 100 mg is not exceeded because the disadvantages are likely to outweigh the advantages.

Epidural anaesthesia (indicated in blue on the partogram) is provided when pethidine does not afford adequate relief, or at an earlier stage should the woman be unduly upset.

PARTOGRAM 7

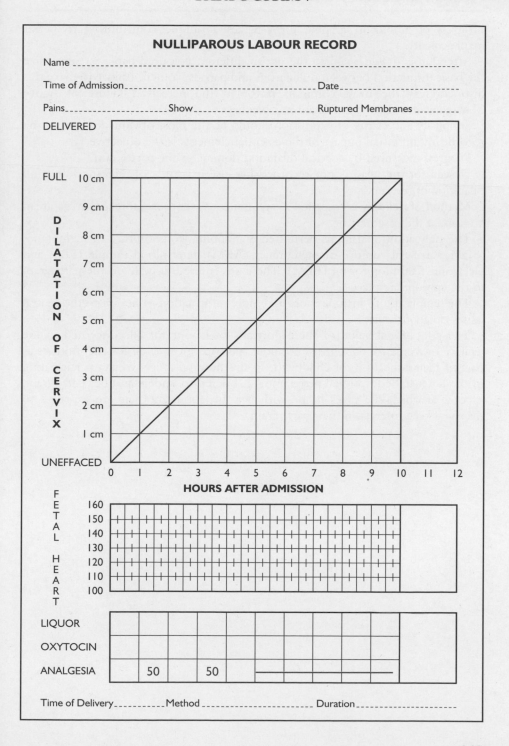

Method of delivery and additional items

Progress of labour in graphic form makes a unique contribution to better management.

Attention is drawn again to the use of different coloured paper to emphasize the basic distinction between nulliparous and parous women. Failure to make this distinction is the most common factor in the perceived failure of Active Management of Labour to attain its objectives.

Simplicity and clarity of expression should be the most obvious features of the record. Instant visual impact of the essential elements is the objective.

Progress measured by cervical dilatation dominates the partogram.

Descent of the head is not recorded because it is only of relevance after full dilatation of the cervix.

Method of delivery is recorded as spontaneous, ventouse, forceps or caesarean section, as the case may be.

The only additional items permitted are: spontaneous rupture of membranes (SRM), artificial rupture of membranes (ARM), fetal blood sample (FBS) and electronic fetal monitoring (EFM). These are entered directly on the partogram in the appropriate place.

The temptation to include more and more information irrelevant to the central issues of labour must be resisted.

The educational value of these portraits of labour for all concerned in the welfare of women in labour is enormous, perhaps most of all for the mothers as part of their education for childbirth. In this hospital every woman participating in the antenatal educational programme is briefed to understand her partogram, a copy of which she takes home with her. In labour mothers are expected to display a keen interest in their partogram.

PARTOGRAM 8

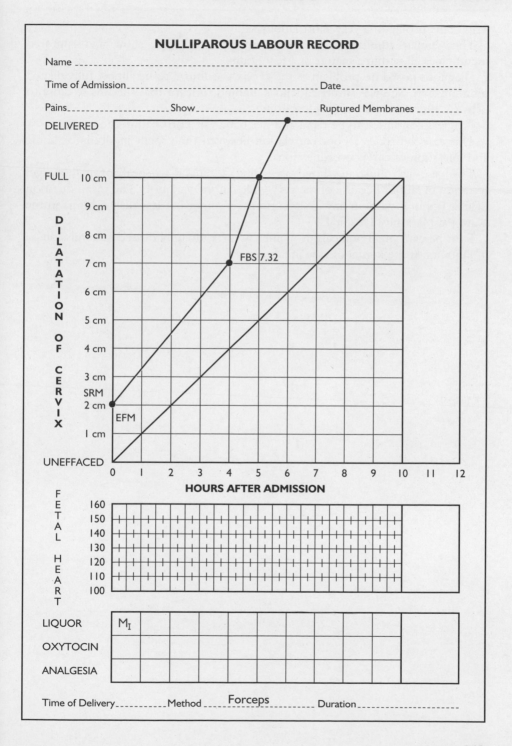

Normal labour (1)

This is the profile of a very short labour.

The woman admitted herself to hospital with pains, show and ruptured membranes all within a matter of a few hours.

Diagnosis posed no problem as the cervix was found to be almost fully dilated on admission. She was surprised, and delighted to learn that she was so close to delivery after such a short period of time.

Progress continued to be rapid and her baby was born within the hour.

This case illustrates a poor correlation between time spent in labour at home and dilatation of cervix on admission.

This case also illustrates how misleading it can be to speak of an 'average' duration of labour because of the very wide natural variation. The mean duration of first labour – without any intervention – is somewhat less than 6 hours in the National Maternity Hospital.

Four percent of all nulliparous women are already fully dilated at admission.

Duration is the kernel of care in labour.

PARTOGRAM 9

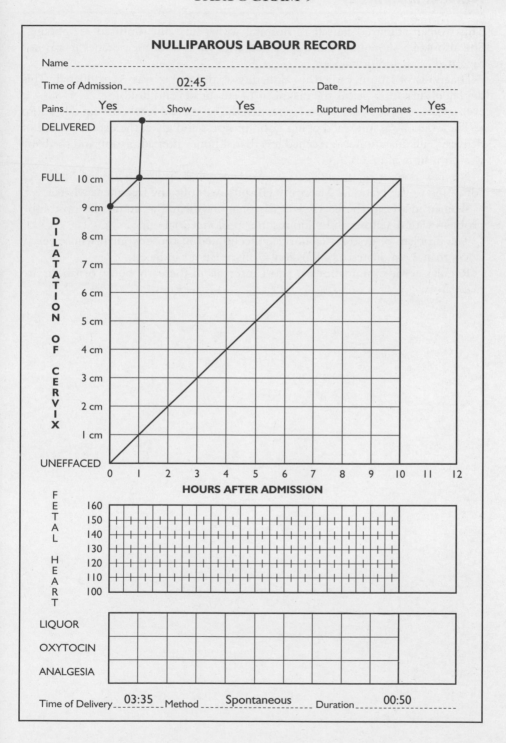

NULLIPAROUS LABOUR RECORD

Name ....

Time of Admission............ 02:45 .... Date........................

Pains........ Yes .... Show............ Yes .... Ruptured Membranes ...... Yes ...

DELIVERED

FULL 10 cm

9 cm

D I L A T A T I O N   O F   C E R V I X

8 cm

7 cm

6 cm

5 cm

4 cm

3 cm

2 cm

1 cm

UNEFFACED

0   1   2   3   4   5   6   7   8   9   10   11   12

HOURS AFTER ADMISSION

F E T A L   H E A R T

160
150
140
130
120
110
100

LIQUOR

OXYTOCIN

ANALGESIA

Time of Delivery........ 03:35 .... Method .... Spontaneous ..... Duration........... 00:50 ...

Normal labour (2)

This woman admitted herself to hospital with pains and ruptured membranes. She also had a show but as this appeared after rupture of membranes it was not regarded as an additional sign.

Diagnosis of labour caused no difficulty as the cervix was 3 cm dilated. This degree of dilatation places the diagnosis of labour beyond doubt.

Progress was assessed 2 hours later when the cervix had reached 7 cm dilatation.

The woman was informed of her good progress and given the expected time of delivery. Full dilatation was reached less than 4 hours after admission and the baby was born soon after.

No less than 40% of nulliparous women are delivered within 4 hours of admission to the National Maternity Hospital without any treatment whatsoever.

Women in whom the cervix is 2 cm or more dilated at admission pose little problem with diagnosis and seldom suffer prolonged labour.

The problem of dystocic labour is concentrated in those women whose cervix is less than 2 cm dilated at admission, or have labour induced.

Regular pelvic examinations at short intervals in the early hours of labour are mandatory.

PARTOGRAM 10

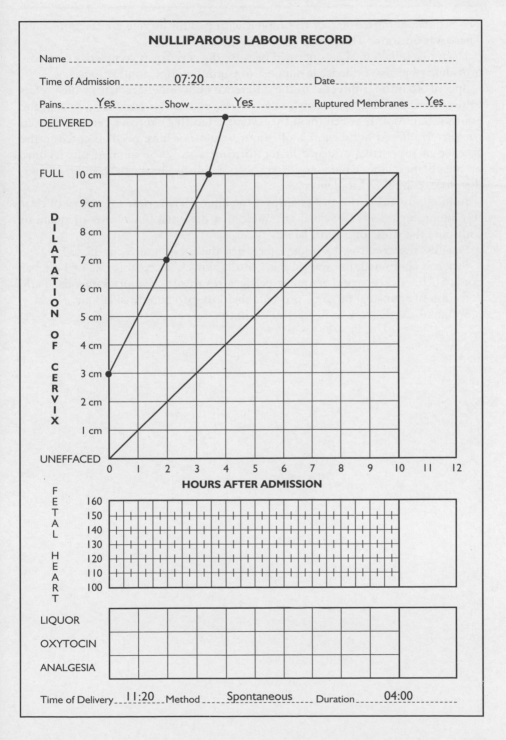

NULLIPAROUS LABOUR RECORD

Name ....

Time of Admission .... 07:20 .... Date ....

Pains .... Yes .... Show .... Yes .... Ruptured Membranes ... Yes ...

DELIVERED

FULL   10 cm

D I L A T A T I O N   O F   C E R V I X

9 cm

8 cm

7 cm

6 cm

5 cm

4 cm

3 cm

2 cm

1 cm

UNEFFACED

0 1 2 3 4 5 6 7 8 9 10 11 12

HOURS AFTER ADMISSION

F E T A L   H E A R T

160
150
140
130
120
110
100

LIQUOR

OXYTOCIN

ANALGESIA

Time of Delivery ..... 11:20 ... Method ..... Spontaneous ..... Duration .... 04:00 ......

Normal labour (3)

This woman admitted herself to hospital with painful uterine contractions only. There was no show. The membranes were intact.

Diagnosis of labour was confirmed because the cervix was completely effaced – providing objective evidence in support of painful uterine contractions.

Special attention is directed to the difference between effacement, which refers to the canal, and dilatation which refers to the external os and, in particular, the point of transition between these two events. Had this woman's cervix not been completely effaced her diagnosis of labour would not have been accepted in the absence of supportive evidence in the form of a show or spontaneous rupture of membranes. She would not have been retained in the labour ward and, therefore, committed to delivery.

Amniotomy was performed to inspect the liquor. There was a free flow of clear (C) liquor, regarded as a virtual guarantee that placental function is adequate to withstand the stress of normal labour.

Progress was confirmed 2 hours later when the cervix was 3 cm dilated.

Progress continued, but was sluggish, at the slowest acceptable rate of 1 cm per hour. Such cases demand frequent pelvic assessments at short intervals. Early detection of abnormal progress prevents the drift into abnormal labour.

Spontaneous delivery took place at 10 hours.

PARTOGRAM 11

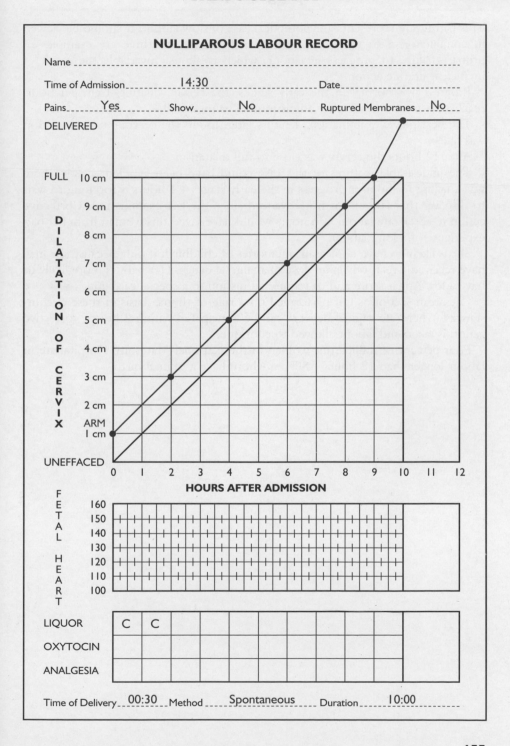

NULLIPAROUS LABOUR RECORD

Name _____

Time of Admission _____ 14:30 _____ Date _____

Pains _____ Yes _____ Show _____ No _____ Ruptured Membranes ___ No ___

DELIVERED

FULL   10 cm

**D
I
L
A
T
A
T
I
O
N

O F

C
E
R
V
I
X**

9 cm
8 cm
7 cm
6 cm
5 cm
4 cm
3 cm
2 cm
ARM
1 cm

UNEFFACED

0   1   2   3   4   5   6   7   8   9   10   11   12

HOURS AFTER ADMISSION

**F
E
T
A
L

H
E
A
R
T**

160
150
140
130
120
110
100

LIQUOR | C | C

OXYTOCIN

ANALGESIA

Time of Delivery __ 00:30 __ Method _____ Spontaneous _____ Duration _____ 10:00

Abnormal labour: slow progress (1)

This partogram represents a hypothetical case of slow labour. It should be viewed in conjunction with the two profiles which follow. All three are examples of primary failure to progress in labour, which is almost invariably the result of inefficient uterine action.

Progress was normal in the early stages: the cervix, dilating 1 cm per hour, reached 4 cm at 3 hours after admission; all seemed well.

The next pelvic examination, 4 hours later, found the cervix 6 cm. No action was taken.

After 12 hours the cervix was close to full dilatation.

The undesirable features of this case could have been avoided. Firstly, there was a failure to monitor progress in the early stages – 4 hours is too long to wait to discover that labour has not advanced since the last examination. Corrective action to accelerate labour at 6 hours would have saved this woman from her bad experience of a long labour.

She is likely to have unpleasant memories of childbirth if only because she may have received a relatively large dose of analgesic drugs. Her baby is more likely to have a low Apgar score and to require admission to a special care unit.

Caesarean section is not performed on a rule-of-thumb basis in these circumstances. When safe vaginal delivery can be anticipated within 2 hours, corrective action is taken and labour allowed to continue.

Four percent of nulliparous women in the National Maternity Hospital are in labour longer than 12 hours – 80% of whom have a vaginal birth.

PARTOGRAM 12

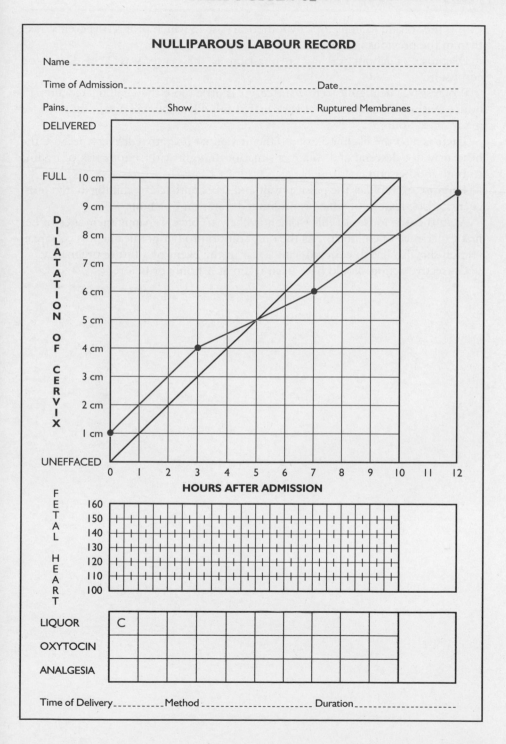

Abnormal labour: slow progress (2)

This is the second example of a hypothetical case in which progress is even slower than in the previous instance.

Diagnosis of labour was not in question as the cervix was 2 cm dilated on admission.

Progress was negligible so that the cervix is little more than half dilated after 12 hours. In these circumstances it is clear that full dilatation will not be attained for many more hours.

There is also the likelihood of a difficult vaginal operative delivery because the head may not descend and rotate, a situation fraught with serious risk of trauma to both mother and child.

This case exemplifies the passive 'wait and see' approach to childbirth, the most characteristic feature of which is prolonged duration of labour.

As in the previous case this woman is likely to have unhappy memories of her first experience of childbirth. As the only solution to her predicament is caesarean section she also has to contend with a scar in the event of a future pregnancy.

Corrective action should have been taken at 4 hours or before.

PARTOGRAM 13

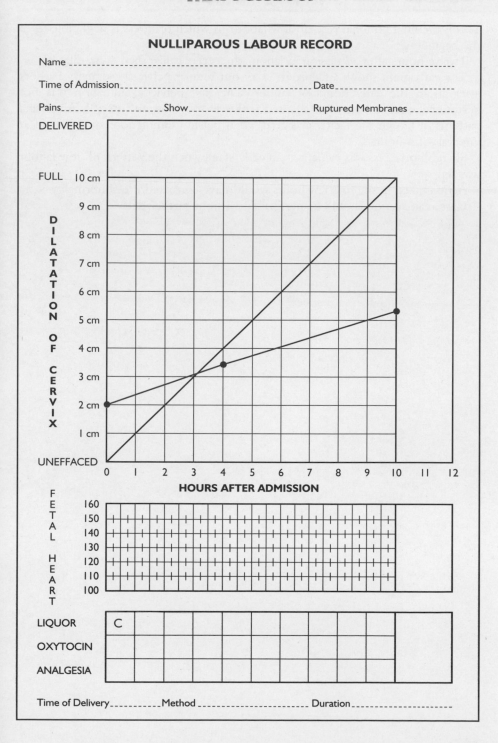

Abnormal labour: slow progress (3)

This is the final notional case of slow labour in which progress is negligible from the beginning.

Twelve hours after admission in labour the cervix is less than 4 cm dilated.

The partogram shows a failure to carry out regular pelvic assessments at short intervals in the early hours of labour. The first pelvic examination was not performed until 4 hours had elapsed – this is too long an interval. Abnormal patterns of labour are tacitly accepted when pelvic examination is performed at intervals of 4 hours.

Sluggish progress was evident at an early stage when the pattern of slow labour was set.

Action taken in the first few hours would have corrected the abnormality.

Caesarean section should be performed without further delay.

PARTOGRAM 14

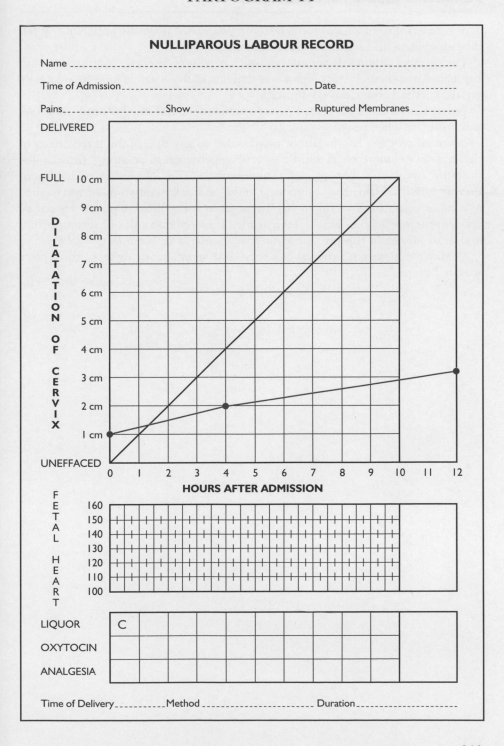

NULLIPAROUS LABOUR RECORD

Name _____

Time of Admission_____ Date_____

Pains_____ Show_____ Ruptured Membranes _____

DELIVERED

FULL 10 cm

D I L A T A T I O N   O F   C E R V I X

9 cm
8 cm
7 cm
6 cm
5 cm
4 cm
3 cm
2 cm
1 cm

UNEFFACED

0 1 2 3 4 5 6 7 8 9 10 11 12

HOURS AFTER ADMISSION

F E T A L   H E A R T

160
150
140
130
120
110
100

LIQUOR   C

OXYTOCIN

ANALGESIA

Time of Delivery_____ Method _____ Duration_____

Abnormal labour: secondary arrest (1)

This is an example of a case in which labour proceeded normally until close on full dilatation when no further progress was made.

The woman admitted herself because of painful uterine contractions and rupture of membranes; clear liquor was draining. Pelvic examination found a fully effaced cervix. Labour was confirmed.

Progress, assessed by repeated pelvic examination, was normal until the cervix reached 8 cm when progress came to a halt.

Arrest of progress late in labour may be due to any one of the three causes of dystocia, but is more characteristic of cephalopelvic disproportion – or occipito-posterior position – than of inefficient uterine action. Nevertheless, inefficient uterine action remains the commonest cause and delay must not be ascribed to any other cause until oxytocin has been given for a limited period to ensure efficient uterine action. This treatment identifies genuine cases of disproportion and bears no risk of rupture of the nulliparous uterus or harm to the baby.

Oxytocin was given; progress resumed and spontaneous delivery took place within 2 hours.

PARTOGRAM 15

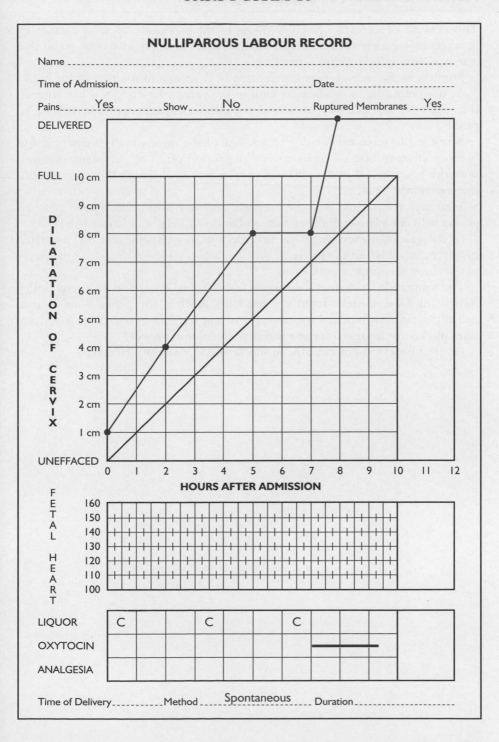

NULLIPAROUS LABOUR RECORD

Name _____

Time of Admission _____ Date _____

Pains _____ Yes _____ Show _____ No _____ Ruptured Membranes _____ Yes ____

DELIVERED

FULL

DILATATION OF CERVIX

10 cm
9 cm
8 cm
7 cm
6 cm
5 cm
4 cm
3 cm
2 cm
1 cm

UNEFFACED

0 1 2 3 4 5 6 7 8 9 10 11 12

HOURS AFTER ADMISSION

FETAL HEART

160
150
140
130
120
110
100

LIQUOR | C | | C | | C | | |
OXYTOCIN
ANALGESIA

Time of Delivery _____ Method _____ Spontaneous _____ Duration _____

Abnormal labour: secondary arrest (2)

This example of secondary arrest is similar to the previous case, with satisfactory progress in the early stages, except, in this instance, labour does not come to a standstill until full dilatation is reached.

Progress in the second stage is measured by descent and rotation of the head.

At this point, the baby's head is high in the pelvis, the occiput is not rotated, the vagina has not been stretched and the mother experiences no inclination to push.

Arrest at this stage may be due to any one of the three causes of dystocia, but is more characteristic of cephalopelvic disproportion – or persistent occipito-posterior position – than of inefficient uterine action, although the latter remains the commonest cause.

Treatment is the same as in the previous case: oxytocin is infused for a limited period with complete confidence that no harm will befall mother or baby.

In this case, however, there was no response to oxytocin, and the unrotated head remained high in the pelvis.

Caesarean section was performed.

The temptation to attempt delivery by traction simply because the cervix is fully dilated must be resisted. Until the head has reached the pelvic floor, vaginal delivery entails instrumental rotation and strong traction to overcome soft tissue resistance. Serious vaginal trauma is not an uncommon result.

Keilland forceps is not available in the National Maternity Hospital.

PARTOGRAM 16

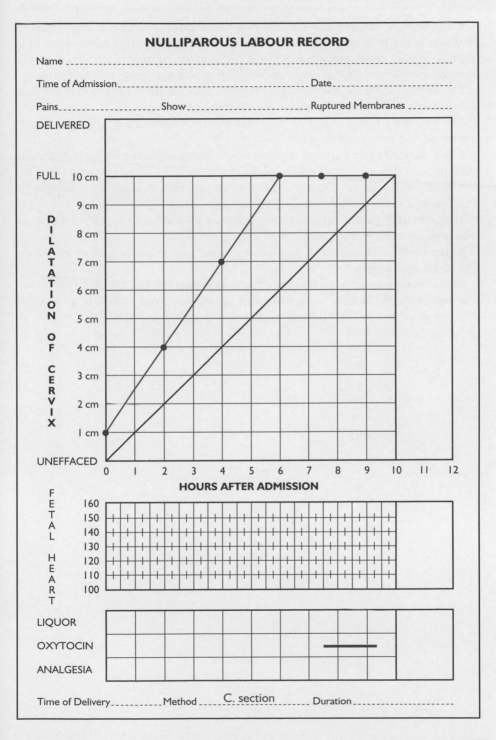

NULLIPAROUS LABOUR RECORD

Name ....

Time of Admission .... Date ....

Pains .... Show .... Ruptured Membranes ....

DELIVERED

FULL

DILATATION OF CERVIX

10 cm
9 cm
8 cm
7 cm
6 cm
5 cm
4 cm
3 cm
2 cm
1 cm

UNEFFACED

0 1 2 3 4 5 6 7 8 9 10 11 12

HOURS AFTER ADMISSION

FETAL HEART

160
150
140
130
120
110
100

LIQUOR

OXYTOCIN

ANALGESIA

Time of Delivery .... Method .... C. section .... Duration ....

Method of treatment: artificial rupture of membranes

Artificial rupture of membranes is performed in all cases as soon as a firm diagnosis of labour is made. This procedure is carried out in the delivery unit only and if there is doubt about the diagnosis the decision to rupture the membranes is deferred for 1 hour; rupturing the membranes is not a decision taken lightly.

The nature of the liquor provides vital evidence of the baby's condition and therefore it should be inspected at an early stage of labour.

The first suspicion of impaired placental function often arises when the liquor is released and meconium is seen.

A free flow of clear liquor is regarded as valuable evidence of good placental function.

Absence of liquor or a heavy suspension of meconium raises the question of fetal hypoxia.

The practice of early rupture of membranes also affords the opportunity to anticipate prolapse of the cord.

In the event of slow labour, amniotomy alone may improve uterine efficiency and accelerate progress.

In no circumstances is oxytocin used when the membranes are intact.

Spontaneous rupture of membranes has already occurred in 30% of all women who admit themselves to hospital in the belief that they are in labour.

PARTOGRAM 17

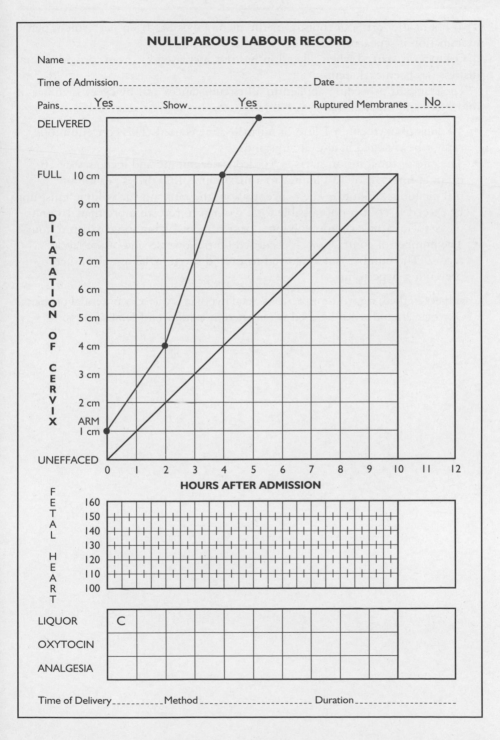

NULLIPAROUS LABOUR RECORD

Name _____

Time of Admission _____ Date _____

Pains _____ Yes _____ Show _____ Yes _____ Ruptured Membranes ___ No ___

DELIVERED

FULL   10 cm

9 cm

D
I   8 cm
L
A   7 cm
T
A   6 cm
T
I   5 cm
O
N   4 cm

O F   3 cm

C   2 cm
E
R   ARM
V   1 cm
I
X
UNEFFACED

0   1   2   3   4   5   6   7   8   9   10   11   12

HOURS AFTER ADMISSION

F   160
E   150
T   140
A   130
L   120
H   110
E   100
A
R
T

LIQUOR   C

OXYTOCIN

ANALGESIA

Time of Delivery _____ Method _____ Duration _____

Method of treatment: oxytocin infusion (1)

Two hours after artificial rupture of the membranes has been performed, pelvic examination is repeated.

Oxytocin is started when dilatation has not increased by 2 cm, provided fetal distress has been excluded.

The standard procedure applied in all circumstances and by every member of midwifery and medical staff is as follows:

- 10 units of oxytocin in 1 litre of normal saline is used. This concentration cannot be changed in any circumstances.
- The rate of the infusion starts at 10 drops per minute and increases by 10 drops at intervals of 15 minutes to a maximum of 60 drops per minute (40 milliunits/minute). The concentration, the rate and the volume must not be exceeded, so it is not possible for a woman to receive more than 10 units of oxytocin, 1 litre of normal saline, or treatment lasting longer than 6 hours.
- The number of contractions is recorded on the reverse side of the labour record. The number is not allowed to exceed seven in 15 minutes, thereby preventing hypertonus.

Subject to these rigorous restrictions, fetal hypoxia is the only potential problem. Oxytocin should *never* be used when there is evidence of fetal distress.

PARTOGRAM 18

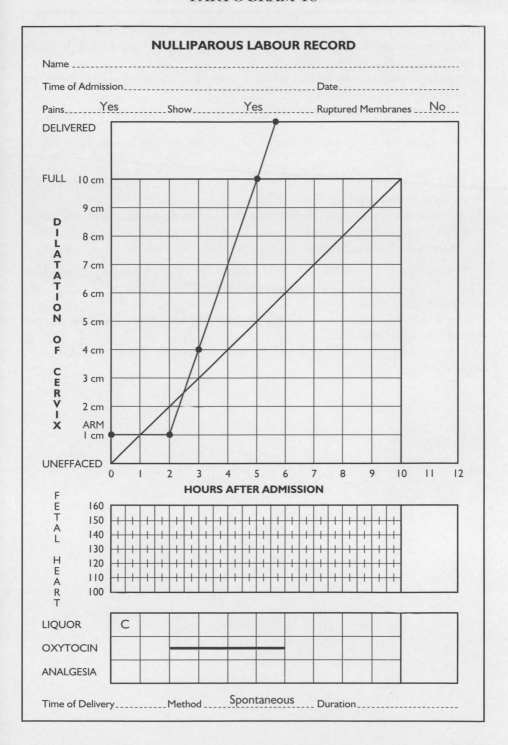

NULLIPAROUS LABOUR RECORD

Name _____

Time of Admission _____ Date _____

Pains _____ Yes _____ Show _____ Yes _____ Ruptured Membranes ___ No ___

DELIVERED

DILATATION OF CERVIX

FULL — 10 cm
9 cm
8 cm
7 cm
6 cm
5 cm
4 cm
3 cm
2 cm
ARM — 1 cm
UNEFFACED

0 1 2 3 4 5 6 7 8 9 10 11 12
HOURS AFTER ADMISSION

FETAL HEART
160
150
140
130
120
110
100

LIQUOR — C

OXYTOCIN

ANALGESIA

Time of Delivery _____ Method _____ Spontaneous _____ Duration _____

Method of treatment: oxytocin infusion (2)

This case illustrates the use of oxytocin in the second stage of labour.

Progress of labour was normal in the first stage, proceeding to full dilatation within a reasonable period of time.

Progress ceased early in the second stage – the head remained high in the pelvis, in an unrotated position.

The mother had no desire to push because there was no pressure on her pelvic floor.

The vagina was, of course, undilated because the woman was in phase one of the second stage.

There were three options in treatment:

- rotation and delivery
- caesarean section to avoid the likelihood of a difficult rotation and delivery through an undilated vagina
- oxytocin for a limited period of time.

The last option was taken, and the standard oxytocin infusion was commenced. This resulted in descent and rotation of the head, thus avoiding a difficult and potentially dangerous delivery.

Should the head not reach the pelvic floor within 1 hour, caesarean section would have been performed.

Oxytocin can be an invaluable aid in the management of slow progress in the second stage.

PARTOGRAM 19

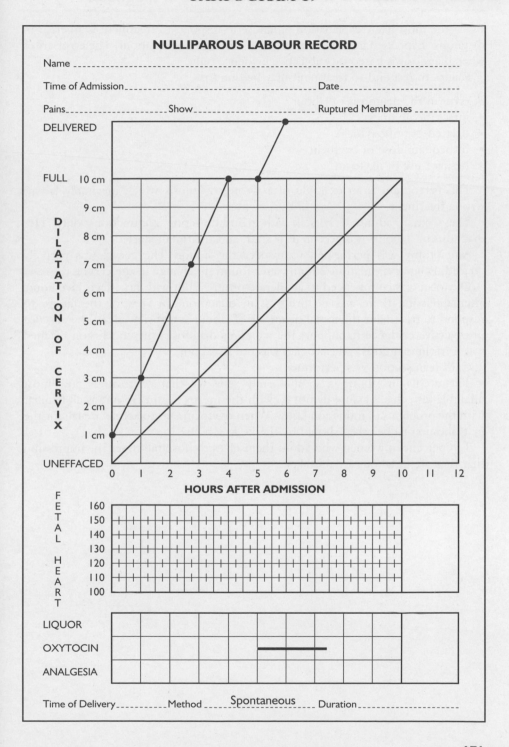

NULLIPAROUS LABOUR RECORD

Name ....

Time of Admission .... Date ....

Pains .... Show .... Ruptured Membranes ....

DELIVERED

FULL

DILATATION OF CERVIX

10 cm
9 cm
8 cm
7 cm
6 cm
5 cm
4 cm
3 cm
2 cm
1 cm

UNEFFACED

0   1   2   3   4   5   6   7   8   9   10   11   12

HOURS AFTER ADMISSION

FETAL HEART

160
150
140
130
120
110
100

LIQUOR

OXYTOCIN

ANALGESIA

Time of Delivery .... Method ...... Spontaneous ...... Duration ....

171

Failure to respond to treatment: error in diagnosis

By far the most likely explanation of failure to respond to treatment is an error in diagnosis. Expressed in simple terms, the woman is not in labour. The error arises when diagnosis is based on subjective evidence only.

Failure to respond to treatment may be due to:

- error in the diagnosis of labour
- intact membranes
- delayed use of oxytocin
- inadequate dose of oxytocin
- hesitant use of oxytocin.

This partogram is an example of a wrong diagnosis which inevitably led to wrong treatment.

The woman admitted herself with painful uterine contractions only. Her diagnosis of 'labour' was accepted by staff, and treatment started.

Amniotomy was performed to inspect the liquor. The cervix was partially effaced. Pelvic examination 2 hours later found no change in the cervix.

Oxytocin was commenced to accelerate progress but with no effect. Five hours after admission there was no progress in dilatation. In view of the failure to respond to treatment the initial diagnosis of labour was reviewed. In the absence of objective evidence to support the woman's diagnosis, the conclusion reached was error in diagnosis – the woman was not in labour.

Caesarean section was performed.

The uterus in labour is so uniformly sensitive that oxytocin is an almost infallible test; this is assuredly not so with the uterus not in labour, as all familiar with the problems of induction know. When oxytocin fails to accelerate labour the first question to be asked should be 'Is she in labour?'.

Ten percent of women who admit themselves to hospital under the impression that they are in labour are mistaken.

PARTOGRAM 20

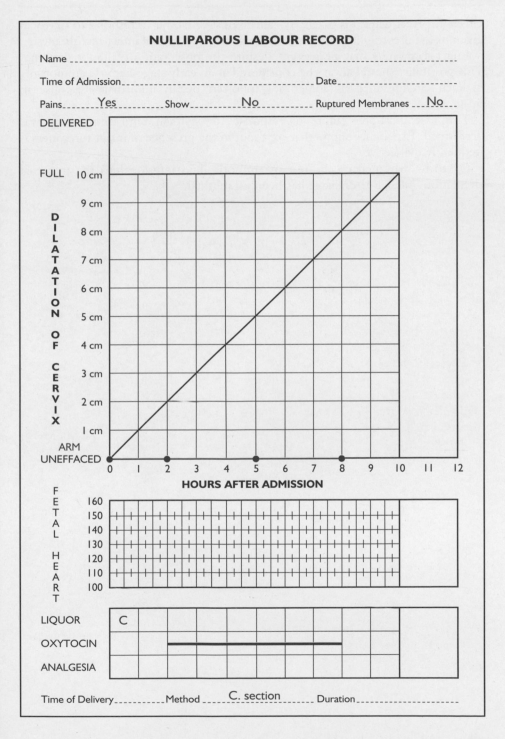

NULLIPAROUS LABOUR RECORD

Name _____

Time of Admission _____ Date _____

Pains _____ Yes _____ Show _____ No _____ Ruptured Membranes ___ No ___

DELIVERED

D I L A T A T I O N   O F   C E R V I X

FULL 10 cm
9 cm
8 cm
7 cm
6 cm
5 cm
4 cm
3 cm
2 cm
1 cm
ARM UNEFFACED

0 1 2 3 4 5 6 7 8 9 10 11 12

HOURS AFTER ADMISSION

F E T A L   H E A R T
160
150
140
130
120
110
100

LIQUOR   C

OXYTOCIN

ANALGESIA

Time of Delivery _____ Method _____ C. section _____ Duration _____

Failure to respond to treatment: membranes intact

Given a correct diagnosis of labour, failure of slow labour to respond to oxytocin given in the prescribed manner should raise the question of intact membranes.

Intact forewaters may be present despite the observation of liquor draining. This possibility should always be considered at an early stage because amniotomy in such circumstances is sometimes followed by an immediate response in progress.

This case illustrates failure of response to oxytocin until amniotomy was performed. Experience shows that oxytocin in the presence of intact forewaters is frequently ineffective.

Oxytocin may increase the risk of amniotic fluid infusion into the maternal circulation unless free drainage has been established.

PARTOGRAM 21

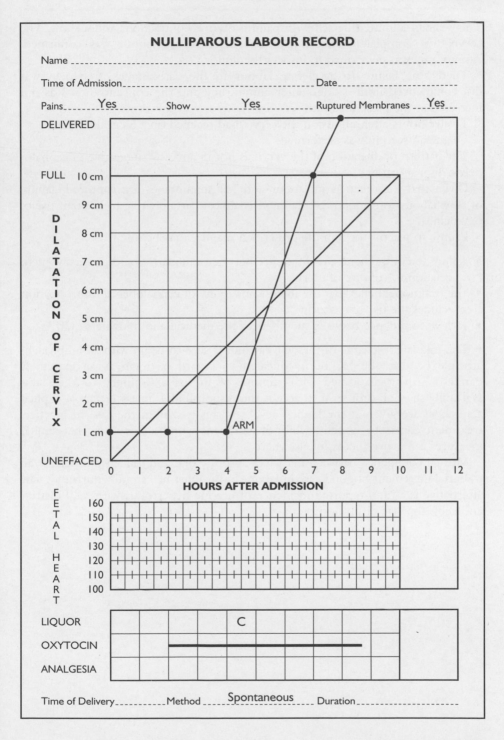

Failure to respond to treatment: hesitant use of oxytocin

This woman admitted herself with painful uterine contractions and a show. The cervix was completely effaced and her diagnosis of labour was confirmed. Amniotomy was performed to inspect the liquor.

There was failure to accelerate labour in the early stages. Oxytocin was not commenced until 5 hours after amniotomy and the concentration was not increased at the prescribed rate.

Twelve hours after admission the cervix had reached only 5 cm dilatation.

Caesarean section was performed.

The pattern of dilatation of the cervix is not in any way suggestive of cephalo-pelvic disproportion.

Given that a woman is in labour and her membranes are ruptured, failure of slow labour to respond to treatment is almost certainly due to hesitant use of oxytocin.

Failure to use oxytocin in the prescribed manner may be due to:

- failure to comprehend the difference between nulliparous and parous women in relation to rupture of uterus
- the traditional belief that the merest possibility of cephalopelvic disproportion precludes the use of oxytocin
- lack of confidence between members of the medical and midwifery staff.

The midwife in charge of the delivery unit is sure to begin with an ambivalent attitude because she has been educated to regard oxytocin as an extremely dangerous drug associated with rupture of uterus and injury to the baby. Naturally she does not wish to accept the responsibility unless the most explicit assurances are given at the highest level. As this is seldom the case in practice, treatment comes to nought, while obstetricians wonder how it is that similar measures can prove successful elsewhere.

Mutual confidence between midwives and doctors, and indeed mothers, is an essential ingredient of good care in labour but it must be carefully nurtured. The alternative is a high reported incidence of uterine hypertonus with fetal distress and cephalopelvic disproportion.

PARTOGRAM 22

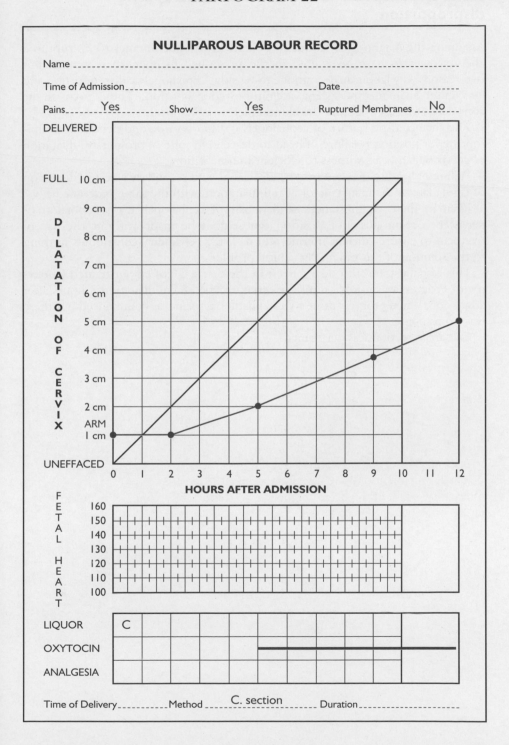

NULLIPAROUS LABOUR RECORD

Name _____

Time of Admission _____ Date _____

Pains _____ Yes _____ Show _____ Yes _____ Ruptured Membranes ____ No ____

DELIVERED

FULL 10 cm

DILATATION OF CERVIX

9 cm
8 cm
7 cm
6 cm
5 cm
4 cm
3 cm
2 cm
ARM
1 cm

UNEFFACED

0 1 2 3 4 5 6 7 8 9 10 11 12

HOURS AFTER ADMISSION

FETAL HEART

160
150
140
130
120
110
100

LIQUOR   C

OXYTOCIN

ANALGESIA

Time of Delivery _____ Method _____ C. section _____ Duration _____

Failure to respond to treatment: cephalopelvic disproportion

Assuming the diagnosis of labour to be correct, the membranes to be ruptured and oxytocin to have been used in the prescribed manner, there remain but two reasons why labour may continue to be slow: cephalopelvic disproportion and its clinical analogue, persistent occipitoposterior position. These two can be considered together because the clinical picture is identical.

The characteristic feature of cephalopelvic disproportion and persistent occipitoposterior position is failure of head to descend in spite of progressive dilatation of cervix which bears witness to efficient uterine action.

Failure of head to descend may be associated with secondary arrest in dilatation of cervix late in the first stage or at full dilatation, with the same outcome.

Even in these circumstances a diagnosis of cephalopelvic disproportion or persistent occipitoposterior position can seldom be made without the use of oxytocin to ensure efficient uterine action. X-ray pelvimetry contributes nothing to the solution of this essentially clinical problem.

This case illustrates secondary arrest in the first stage of labour treated by oxytocin. Progress was normal until the cervix reached 8 cm dilatation 5 hours after admission. When progress came to a standstill oxytocin was commenced but there was no response.

Caesarean section was performed.

PARTOGRAM 23

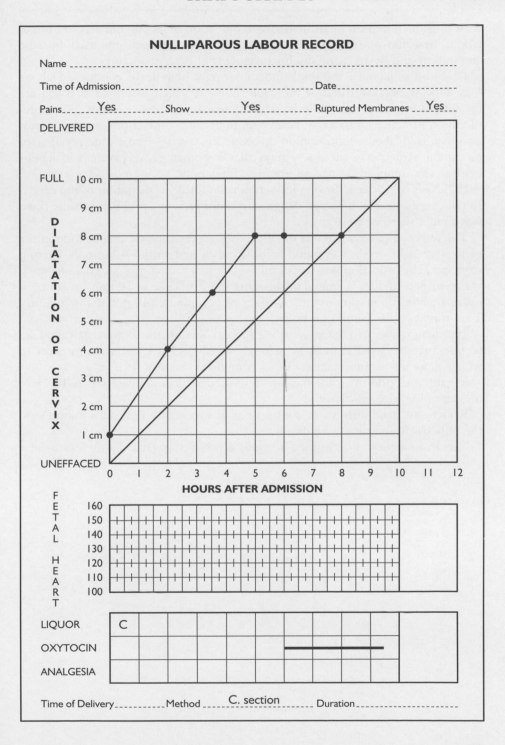

NULLIPAROUS LABOUR RECORD

Name _____

Time of Admission _____ Date _____

Pains _____ Yes _____ Show _____ Yes _____ Ruptured Membranes ___ Yes ___

DELIVERED

FULL 10 cm

DILATATION OF CERVIX

9 cm

8 cm

7 cm

6 cm

5 cm

4 cm

3 cm

2 cm

1 cm

UNEFFACED

0 1 2 3 4 5 6 7 8 9 10 11 12

HOURS AFTER ADMISSION

FETAL HEART

160
150
140
130
120
110
100

LIQUOR   C

OXYTOCIN

ANALGESIA

Time of Delivery _____ Method _____ C. section _____ Duration _____

Induction: success

A clear distinction must be made between induction of labour and acceleration of labour that has already begun. Confusion exists between the two because amniotomy and oxytocin are essential elements of both procedures.

Diagnosis of labour – the single most important item in the conduct of labour – is difficult because three of the four signs on which diagnosis is based are invalidated by the process of induction: ruptured membranes, show and painful uterine contractions. Oxytocin causes painful uterine contractions whether or not a woman is in labour; confusion on this issue has given rise to a widespread error in clinical obstetrics – the assumption that a woman on oxytocin is in labour because she complains of painful uterine contractions.

Diagnosis of labour following induction rests solely on dilatation of the cervix. In the case illustrated, however, diagnosis did not present a problem because there was a rapid response to oxytocin.

The response to oxytocin was monitored by repeated pelvic examination in the early stages; the cervix was found to be 3 cm dilated within 4 hours of starting oxytocin. The induction was successful.

Oxytocin to induce is limited to the same standard dose of 10 units in 1 litre of normal saline at a maximum rate of 60 drops per minute (40 milliunits/minute). This imposes a time limit of 6 hours.

The temptation to continue with a second litre in the hope that caesarean section may be avoided must be strongly resisted. These are circumstances in which water intoxication, among other complications, may occur.

Intrauterine pressure catheters are not used. Cervical dilatation is the sole measure of uterine efficiency.

Evidence of fetal distress, or contractions in excess of seven in 15 minutes are the only bar to increasing the drip rate.

Caesarean section is performed if labour is not well advanced after 8 hours.

PARTOGRAM 24

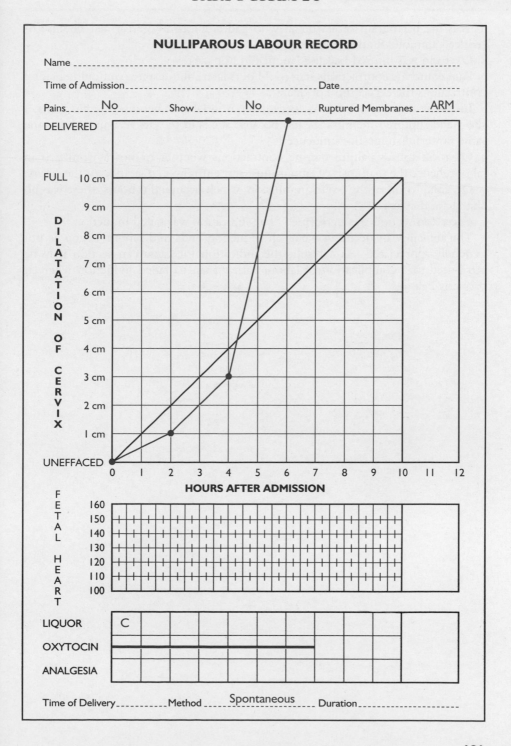

Induction: failure (1)

This is the partogram of a woman who had amniotomy performed because of reduced amniotic fluid volume.

Oxytocin was infused because labour did not start.

Painful uterine contractions started 2 hours later, but despite continuing painful contractions the cervix did not dilate.

In this situation a woman reacts as if she is in labour, because she has pains, a show and ruptured membranes and because she is in the delivery unit under the same powerful suggestive influences.

Oxytocin causes painful uterine contractions whether or not a woman is in labour, hence the diagnosis of labour must rest entirely on dilatation of the cervix.

On completion of the oxytocin infusion, which occupied 6 hours, there was no change in the cervix.

Caesarean section was performed. The indication was failed induction.

The difficulty in deciding when an induction ends and labour begins is not generally appreciated. As a result, the indication for caesarean section may be attributed to a complication of labour rather than to failed induction where it properly belongs.

PARTOGRAM 25

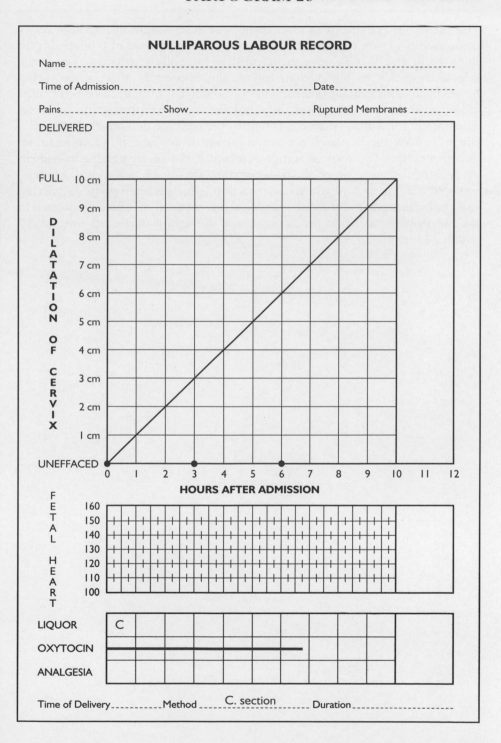

NULLIPAROUS LABOUR RECORD

Name _____

Time of Admission _____ Date _____

Pains _____ Show _____ Ruptured Membranes _____

DELIVERED

FULL   10 cm

9 cm

D   8 cm
I
L   7 cm
A
T   6 cm
A
T   5 cm
I
O   4 cm
N
        3 cm
O
F   2 cm

C   1 cm
E
R
V
I
X

UNEFFACED

    0   1   2   3   4   5   6   7   8   9   10   11   12

HOURS AFTER ADMISSION

F   160
E   150
T   140
A
L   130
        120
H   110
E   100
A
R
T

LIQUOR | C |

OXYTOCIN

ANALGESIA

Time of Delivery _____ Method _____ C. section _____ Duration _____

Induction: failure (2)

This is another example of an unsuccessful case where slight dilatation of cervix took place as a result of stimulation by oxytocin over a period of 6 hours. It is in this type of case that an error in diagnosis is most likely to occur. The cervix reluctantly yields to stimulation, giving the impression that it was being forced open – but genuine dilatation has not occurred. Also, in this type of failed induction there is a temptation to record the indication for section under an all-embracing heading – dystocia, failure to progress, or dubious fetal distress – when in reality the woman was never in labour. Every case of induction subsequently delivered by caesarean section is recorded as a failure because individuals are selected for induction on the basis that they are suitable for vaginal delivery.

There is an alternative to caesarean section, which is appropriate in selected cases once the nature of the case is understood: oxytocin may be discontinued in the reasonable expectation that spontaneous labour will start of its own accord within 24 hours.

PARTOGRAM 26

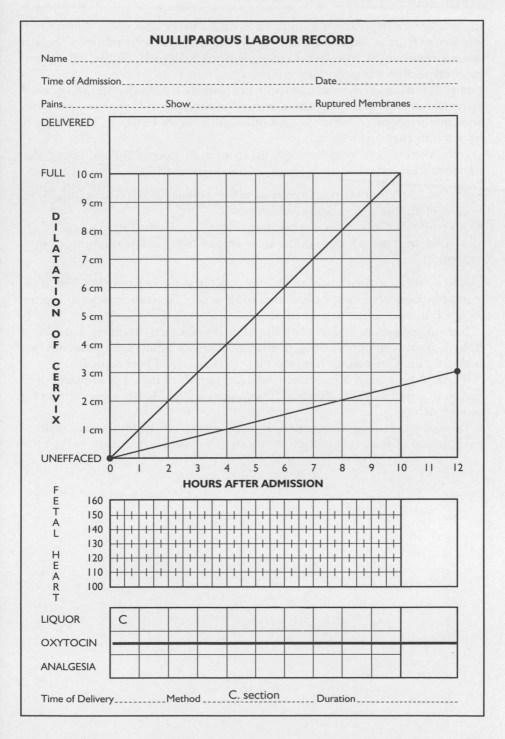

NULLIPAROUS LABOUR RECORD

Name _____

Time of Admission_____ Date_____

Pains_____ Show_____ Ruptured Membranes _____

DELIVERED

FULL   10 cm

D
I
L   9 cm
A
T   8 cm
A
T   7 cm
I
O   6 cm
N
        5 cm
O
F   4 cm

C   3 cm
E
R   2 cm
V
I   1 cm
X

UNEFFACED
        0   1   2   3   4   5   6   7   8   9   10 11 12

HOURS AFTER ADMISSION

F   160
E   150
T   140
A   130
L   120
        110
H   100
E
A
R
T

LIQUOR   C

OXYTOCIN

ANALGESIA

Time of Delivery_____ Method _____ C. section _____ Duration_____

Fetal distress: placental insufficiency/accident of labour

In this case fetal hypoxia was not suspected until a heavy suspension of meconium was seen at routine amniotomy in early labour. The fetal heart rate trace showed late decelerations. A fetal blood sample showed a low pH (7.20) and prompt caesarean section was performed.

Such is the significance attached to meconium as a potential sign of impaired placental function that the practice of routine amniotomy is applied to all cases once the diagnosis of labour is confirmed. Absence of liquor at amniotomy is treated with the same respect.

Fetal distress may occur during the course of normal labour under two circumstances:

- Placental function is already impaired before labour begins as seen typically in cases of intrauterine growth retardation.
- An accident of labour such as prolapse of cord or placental separation. Meconium is not a feature of the acute type of hypoxia that results from an accident.

A fetus with impaired placental function tolerates labour badly. The first suspicion of hypoxia often arises when meconium is seen; meconium seldom appears for the first time during normal labour.

Not all meconium is accorded the same significance. There is a world of difference between light staining of a large volume of liquor and meconium that is virtually undiluted which represents, in effect, severe oligohydramnios.

A fetal blood sample is performed in all cases in which there is a suspicious fetal heart rate pattern. Thick, Grade III meconium is regarded as an indication for prompt delivery.

Decisions regarding treatment are rarely based on EFM tracings without confirmation of suspected hypoxia by a fetal blood sample.

PARTOGRAM 27

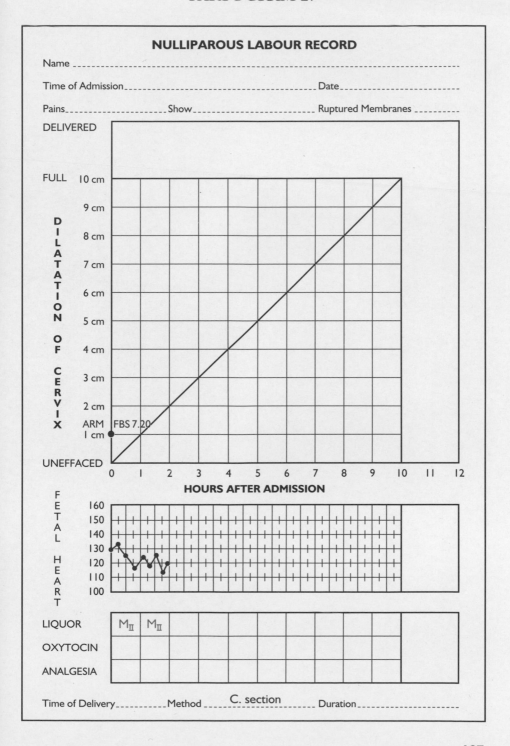

NULLIPAROUS LABOUR RECORD

Name _____

Time of Admission_____ Date_____

Pains_____ Show_____ Ruptured Membranes _____

DELIVERED

FULL   10 cm

9 cm

8 cm

D
I   7 cm
L
A   6 cm
T
A   5 cm
T
I   4 cm
O
N   3 cm

O   2 cm
F
ARM   FBS 7.20
C   1 cm
E
R
V
I
X

UNEFFACED

0   1   2   3   4   5   6   7   8   9   10   11   12

HOURS AFTER ADMISSION

F
E   160
T   150
A   140
L   130
        120
H   110
E   100
A
R
T

LIQUOR M_{II} M_{II}

OXYTOCIN

ANALGESIA

Time of Delivery_____ Method _____ C. section _____ Duration_____

Parous Labour

Parous labour

From the standpoint of labour the parous woman might as well belong to a different biological species, hence the labour record is printed on a different colour paper. Significantly, the sole difference in content is that the word 'Oxytocin' does not appear. Lack of appreciation of the reasons for these distinctions leads to the most prevalent of all obstetric errors: the practice of extrapolating from a first to a subsequent labour. This results in much unnecessary intervention and iatrogenic disorder. There is no basis for comparison as the events are completely unrelated. The salient features of parous labour may be summarized thus:

- The duration, and consequent stress involved, bear no comparison with first labour because the parous woman rarely suffers from inefficient uterine action, and because her genital tract has been stretched before.
- In the event of slow progress another explanation should be sought, the most likely being that she is not in labour.
- Failure to progress in a parous woman who is in labour is often a manifestation of obstruction arising from a fetal cause. This can be easily overlooked with disastrous consequences because the capacity of the pelvis is taken for granted.
- The common cause of obstruction is malpresentation.
- The parous uterus is prone to rupture and this may occur even in the course of normal labour.

Oxytocin should be used to stimulate the parous uterus only after most serious consideration, and on a strictly individual basis. The diagnosis of labour should be reviewed and the causes of obstruction carefully excluded beforehand.

Epidural anaesthesia has little application in the parous woman because one in two can expect to be delivered within 2 hours of admission. Commitment to epidural anaesthesia in a parous woman is based on the false premise that all labours are similar.

PARTOGRAM 28

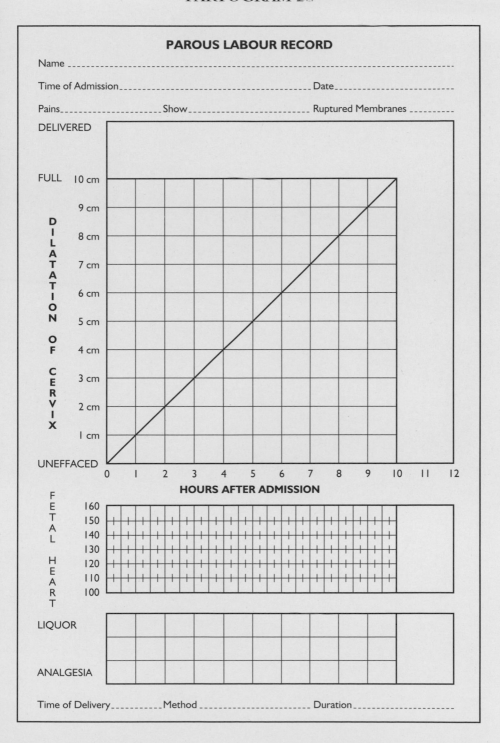

PAROUS LABOUR RECORD

Name _____

Time of Admission _____ Date _____

Pains _____ Show _____ Ruptured Membranes _____

DELIVERED

FULL   10 cm

9 cm

8 cm

D 7 cm
I
L 6 cm
A
T 5 cm
A
T 4 cm
I
O 3 cm
N
2 cm
O F
1 cm
C
E
R UNEFFACED
V   0   1   2   3   4   5   6   7   8   9   10   11   12
I
X   **HOURS AFTER ADMISSION**

F 160
E 150
T 140
A 130
L 120
110
H 100
E
A
R
T

LIQUOR

ANALGESIA

Time of Delivery _____ Method _____ Duration _____

Section III
Clinical Data

Audit of outcome is the framework within which Active Management of Labour is practised.

Clinical data

Table 1 requires little in the way of explanation. As it is part of the philosophy of Active Management of Labour to achieve the best results with the least interference, attention is directed to the following items.

Perinatal mortality rate

Perinatal mortality remains the best objective measure of standards of practice in terms of the child. Notice is drawn to the decrease in the number of postmortem examinations performed. This has special relevance to trauma: in the absence of postmortem examination, death is all too easily attributed to hypoxia.

Caesarean section

In terms of the mother, caesarean section rates serve the same function. The incidence of caesarean section continues to increase and was 14.2% in 2000; there has been no commensurate decrease in perinatal mortality. The caesarean section rate in spontaneously labouring nulliparous women with a single cephalic pregnancy at term (SNSCT)[20] has remained constant, in particular for the indication of dystocia, notwithstanding the increase in the overall caesarean section rate.

Induction

The incidence of induction was 36% in 1970. Thereafter there was a decline when a selective approach to poorly defined risk factors – mainly pre-eclampsia and post-dates pregnancy – was adopted. The induction rate has risen again and was 24.2% in 2000 with no decrease in the perinatal mortality rate.

Vaginal operative delivery

For ease of comparison with other centres, the incidence of vaginal operative deliveries is expressed here as a percentage of total births, whereas in practice some 90% of vaginal operative deliveries were performed in nulliparous women. With the introduction of Active Management of Labour, the incidence of vaginal operative deliveries declined to approximately 6% but now has increased to 11.5%. Rotational forceps deliveries are not carried out in the National Maternity Hospital.

Epidural anaesthesia

There has been a significant increase in epidural anaesthesia since 1990.

Table 1 Comparative figures for 35 years at the National Maternity Hospital

Year	1965	1970	1975	1980	1985	1990	1992	1995	2000
Babies born	5063	6255	7430	8849	7482	6039	6256	6718	7840
Perinatal deaths	185	180	157	126	98	64	57	70	81
Postmortems	181	180	157	122	97	58	53	60	50
Perinatal mortality rate including malformations (per 1000)	36.5	28.8	21.1	14.2	13.1	10.6	9.0	10.4	10.3
Overall caesarean section rate (%)	4.2	4.2	4.1	4.9	5.1	8.5	8.5	10.3	14.2
Caesarean section rate (%) in SNSCT							4.8	5.2	4.8
Induction (%)	28.5	36.0	14.7	13.4	6.7	14.1	11.6	18.5	24.2
Vaginal operative delivery (%)	12.2	7.7	11.0	6.5	5.4	6.5	5.7	9.6	11.5
Epidural anaesthesia (%)						10	31	48	49

SNSCT, spontaneously labouring nulliparous women with a single cephalic pregnancy at term.

Analysis of hospital population

There have been notable changes in the biographical background of the population served in the National Maternity Hospital over the last 35 years. There can be little doubt that many of these changes have contributed to alterations in both the perinatal mortality and caesarean section rates (see *Table 2*).

Maternal age

Maternal age has an important bearing on perinatal mortality. There has been a steady decline in incidence of mothers aged 40 and above, but an increase in incidence of mothers aged 30–39. The number of mothers aged less than 20 reached a peak in the late 1980s and but has started to decrease over the last decade.

Parity

There has been a significant increase in nulliparous women in particular over the last decade with a corresponding decrease of parous women with five or more previous births.

Birth weight

The incidence of low birth weight has remained low, consistently less than 10%. The progressive decline, to 3% in the 1980s, has not continued and has slightly increased over the last decade.

Table 2 Analysis of the hospital population at the National Maternity Hospital (%)

Year	1965	1970	1975	1980	1985	1990	1995	2000
Maternal age								
<20	3	6	8	6	8	9	5	4
20–29	50	58	61	60	55	47	41	37
30–39	39	31	27	32	35	41	51	56
40+	8	5	4	2	2	3	3	3
Parity								
1	26	33	38	35	35	36	41	45
2,3,4	51	51	52	55	57	57	56	55
5+	23	16	10	10	8	7	3	1
Birth weight								
2.5 kg or less	7	6	4	3	3	5	5	5

197

Clinical circumstances of perinatal deaths

Table 3 places perinatal deaths in the clinical context in which they occurred. There were considerable improvements under all headings except one: antenatal care.

By way of contrast, the reductions elsewhere are the more striking because they occurred against the background of an increase in total births.

No antenatal care

The virtual elimination of this category of death reflects the increase in antenatal care.

Antenatal deaths

This category includes late fetal deaths which occurred before the onset of labour. Most were unexplained but intrauterine growth retardation was a common feature. There has been least improvement in this group.

Intrapartum deaths

Apropos the management of labour – the subject of this manual – the improvement that has taken place here needs constant vigilance if it is to be maintained and improved further.

Neonatal deaths

The decrease in this category accounts for the most significant contribution to the improvement in the perinatal mortality rate.

Congenital malformations

The decrease in this category also accounts for a significant contribution to the improvement in perinatal mortality rate.

Table 3 Clinical circumstances of perinatal deaths at the National Maternity Hospital

Year	1965	1970	1975	1980	1985	1990	1995	2000
Total births	5063	6255	7430	8849	7482	6039	6718	7840
No antenatal care	22	16	8	4	0	1	0	0
Antenatal deaths	43	56	70	57	41	26	24	38
Intrapartum deaths	16	24	8	10	11	7	4	4
Neonatal deaths	47	40	38	20	10	8	14	12
Congenital malformations	57	44	33	35	36	22	28	27
Perinatal deaths excluding malformations	128	136	124	93	62	42	42	54
Total deaths	185	180	157	126	98	64	70	81
PNMR total (per 1000)	36.5	28.8	21.1	14.2	10.6	9.0	10.4	10.3
PNMR excluding malformations (per 1000)	25	21.9	16.8	10.6	8.3	7.0	6.3	6.9

PNMR, perinatal mortality rate.

Rupture of uterus

This is the ultimate expression of serious injury to the mother. There was no case of rupture of uterus in more than 100 000 consecutive nulliparous women delivered during a period of 35 years – despite the fact that oxytocin was used in some 40 000 of those nulliparous women to ensure efficient uterine action during labour – and without regard to the possibility of cephalopelvic disproportion.

Dehiscence of a caesarean section scar accounted for 76 of 105 cases of rupture of uterus in parous women.

The confidence necessary to use oxytocin effectively derives ultimately from the information contained in *Table 4* and *Table 5*.

Table 4 Rupture of uterus at the National Maternity Hospital (cumulative figures for the previous 35 years)

Year	1970	1975	1980	1985	1990	1995	2000	Total
Cases	28	17	23	13	7	4	13	105
Nulliparous women	0	0	0	0	0	0	0	0

Traumatic intracranial haemorrhage in firstborn infants

This is the ultimate expression of serious injury to the child.

There were 50 cases of traumatic intracranial haemorrhage in firstborn infants: 26 cephalic and 24 breech presentations. All but four of the 26 cases of traumatic intracranial haemorrhage in firstborn infants with cephalic presentations were vaginal operative deliveries (see *Table 5*).

Traumatic intracranial haemorrhage occurred on four occasions in association with spontaneous vertex delivery in almost 100 000 firstborn infants and in no case was oxytocin used.

This should be read in conjunction with *Table 4*.

Table 5 Traumatic intracranial haemorrhage in firstborn infants at the National Maternity Hospital

Year	1965	1970	1975	1980	1985	1990	1995	2000	Total[a]
Births	1327	2054	2778	3106	2619	2114	2744	3441	93 961
TICH	6	2	4	0	6	1	3	0	50
Breech	2	1	3	0	3	1	0	0	24
Vertex	4	1	1	0	2	0	3	0	26
Vaginal operative delivery of vertex presentation	4	1	1	0	1	0	1	0	22

[a]Cumulative figures for 35 years; nulliparous births.
TICH, traumatic intracranial haemorrhage.

Cerebral dysfunction in mature infants

Permanent brain damage that could have been avoided may well be regarded as the ultimate failure in obstetric practice. So that these may be known and kept under surveillance, all cases of cerebral dysfunction identified in the course of routine examination for this purpose by our neonatologists are placed on record (see *Table 6*).

Cerebral dysfunction is defined as a state of abnormal muscle tone or altered primitive reflexes which occurs in term infants who weigh 2500 g or more. Preterm infants born before 37 completed weeks and infants of low birth weight are specifically excluded.

Hypoxia is clearly the most important factor in this regard, and typically this was the penultimate stage in a process that had existed before labour began – placental insufficiency. Accidents of labour cover prolapse of cord and abruption of placenta. Among the cases of trauma there were six forceps and three breech deliveries. Other causes include drugs, infections and metabolic disorders.

Table 6 Cerebral dysfunction in mature infants in the National Maternity Hospital

Year	1970	1975	1980	1985	1990	1995	2000	Total[a]
Babies born	6255	7430	8849	7482	6039	6718	7840	228 733
Cerebral dysfunction	17	25	29	23	15	7	6	512
Hypoxia	12	17	23	18	11	3	5	374
Accident of labour	3	5	1	2	0	0	0	43
Trauma	0	0	1	1	0	0	0	18
Other causes	2	3	4	2	4	4	1	77

[a] Cumulative figures for 35 years; all births.

Diagnosis of labour

Table 7 lists the evidence with which 1000 consecutive nulliparous women presented at the delivery unit of the National Maternity Hospital in the belief that labour had started.

Some 10% were mistaken, because they failed to pass the initial test of painful uterine contractions. A very high proportion of those who passed this test had the additional evidence of a 'show' or spontaneous rupture of membranes. Notice was taken of a 'show' only when this appeared before the membranes ruptured.

Some with painful uterine contractions had neither of these two signs, in which case the crucial decision as to whether or not to retain was based entirely on complete effacement of cervix.

Table 7 Diagnosis of labour at the National Maternity Hospital in 1000 consecutive nulliparous women

Symptom/sign	%
Pains	89
Show	59
Spontaneous rupture of the membranes	27

Duration of labour in nulliparous women

Duration of labour is synonymous with the time spent in the delivery unit of this hospital before the baby is born: all cases are included, whether or not a state of labour existed initially – a point of special significance in cases of induction.

The mean duration of labour in nulliparous women, without treatment, is somewhat less than 6 hours.

The composite figures given in Table 8 are taken from over 3000 consecutive nulliparous women in 2001. It should be noted that despite the significant increase of epidural anaesthesia, the length of time in labour in nulliparous women has not changed dramatically.

Table 8 Duration of labour in nulliparous women at the National Maternity Hospital in over 3000 consecutive nulliparous women in 2001

Hours	%
<2	13
2–4	16
4–6	20
6–8	22
8–10	16
10–12	9
12+	4
	100

Spontaneously labouring nulliparous women with a single cephalic pregnancy at term

Effacement of the cervix refers to the length of the canal, from above downwards. Dilatation of the cervix refers to the external os only, when effacement is complete. The cervix is not effaced in some 10% and is already fully dilated in some 4% of nulliparous women admitted to the National Maternity Hospital in labour. These two extremes do not relate well with the time spent in labour at home. Rather they are an expression of efficient uterine action as the caesarean section and oxytocin rates in the different groups of women show (see *Table 9* and *Figure III.1*).

Many authors exclude those cases at the lower levels of dilatation and thus exclude the problem cases, both in diagnosis and treatment.

The parous cervix is a different organ altogether.

Table 9 Spontaneously labouring nulliparous women with a single cephalic pregnancy at term, based on a series of 2000 consecutive women from the National Maternity Hospital

Dilatation of cervix	Dilatation of cervix on admission (%)	Caesarean section rate (%)	Oxytocin rate (%)
Not effaced (0 cm)	10	7.0	84
1 cm	43	6.7	69
2 cm	26	4.5	36
3 cm	9	2.4	19
> 4 cm	12	0	12

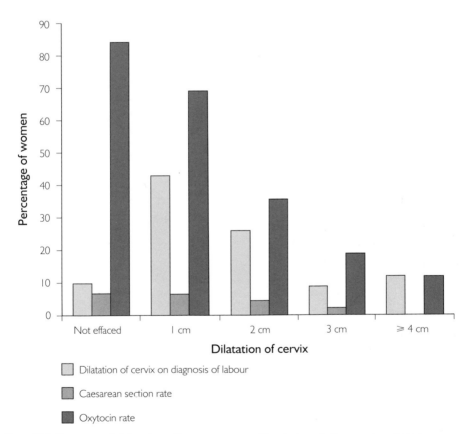

Figure III.1 Spontaneously labouring nulliparous women with a single cephalic pregnancy at term.

Obstetrical norms in nulliparous women

A paradoxical feature of contemporary practice is a steady increase, almost everywhere, in the rate of medical or – more importantly – surgical intervention, despite a remarkable improvement in general health and a precipitous fall in perinatal mortality. There is a widespread tendency to attribute these improved results to this very intervention. Certainly, above anything else, iatrogenic disease – whether physical or emotional – must be avoided.

In conclusion, therefore, particularly in spontaneously labouring nulliparous women with a single cephalic pregnancy at term, it is important to continuously audit all interventions.

What is 'normal' is a difficult issue to address. What is obligatory, though, is knowing the level of interventions, whether they are increasing or decreasing and to have an opinion on whether or not they are appropriate.

References

1 O'Driscoll K, Jackson RJA & Gallagher JT (1969) Prevention of prolonged labour. *British Medical Journal* **ii**: 477–480.
2 O'Driscoll K, Stronge JM & Minogue M (1973) Active management of labour. *British Medical Journal* **iii**: 135–137.
3 O'Driscoll K & Stronge JM (1975) The active management of labour. *Clinics in Obstetrics and Gynaecology* **2**: 3–17.
4 Boylan P & O'Driscoll K (1983) Improvement in perinatal mortality rate attributed to spontaneous preterm labor without use of tocolytic agents. *American Journal of Obstetrics and Gynecology* **145**: 781–783.
5 Boylan P (1976) Oxytocin and neonatal jaundice. *British Medical Journal* **ii**: 564–565.
6 O'Driscoll K, Jackson RJA & Gallagher JT (1970) Active management of labour and cephalopelvic disproportion. *British Journal of Obstetrics and Gynaecology* **77**: 385–389.
7 O'Driscoll K & Stronge JM (1975) Active management of labour and occipito-posterior position. *Australian and New Zealand Journal of Obstetrics and Gynaecology* **15**: 1–4.
8 Daw E (1973) *Journal of Obstetrics and Gynaecology of the British Commonwealth* **80**: 734.
9 O'Driscoll K, Meagher D, MacDonald D & Geoghegan F (1981) Traumatic intracranial haemorrhage in firstborn infants and delivery with obstetric forceps. *British Journal of Obstetrics and Gynaecology* **88**: 577–581.
10 O'Driscoll K (1975) An obstetrician's view of pain. *British Journal of Anaesthesia* **47**: 1053–1059.
11 Impey L, MacQuillan K & Robson MS (2000) Epidural analgesia need not increase operative delivery rates. *American Journal of Obstetrics and Gynecology* **182**: 358–363.
12 O'Driscoll K, Coughlan M, Fenton V & Skelly M (1977) Active management of labour: care of the fetus. *British Medical Journal* **ii**: 1451–1453.
13 MacDonald D, Grant A, Sheridan-Pereira M, Boylan P & Chalmers I (1985) The Dublin randomized controlled trial of intrapartum fetal heart rate monitoring. *American Journal of Obstetrics and Gynecology* **152**: 524–539.
14 Garcia J, Corry M, MacDonald D, Elbourne D & Grant A (1985) Mothers' views of continuous electronic fetal heart monitoring and intermittent auscultation in a randomized controlled trial. *Birth* **12**: 79–85.
15 O'Driscoll K, Carroll CJ & Coughlan M (1975) Selective induction of labour. *British Medical Journal* **iv**: 727–729.
16 O'Driscoll K (1972) Impact of active management on delivery unit practice. *Proceedings of the Royal Society of Medicine* **65**: 697–698.
17 Robson MS (2001) Classification of caesarean sections. *Fetal and Maternal Medicine Review* **12**: 23–39.
18 US Department of Health and Human Services (1981) Public Health Service, National Institutes of Health. Consensus Development Report: *Cesarean Childbirth*. No. 82-2067, October 1981.
19 Grant A, O'Brien N, MacDonald D, Joy MT & Hennessey E (1989) Cerebral palsy among children born during the Dublin randomised trial of intrapartum monitoring. *Lancet* **2**: 1233–1236.
20 National Maternity Hospital (2001) *Annual Clinical Report*. National Maternity Hospital, Dublin, Ireland; pp.113–115.

Further reading

Bottoms SF, Rosen MG & Dokol RJ (1980) The increase in the cesarean birth rate. *New England Journal of Medicine* **302**: 559–562.
Fitzpatrick M & O'Herlihy C (2001) The effects of labour and delivery on the pelvic floor (review). *Best Practice and Research: Clinical Obstetrics and Gynaecology* **15**(1): 63–79.
Fitzpatrick M, McQuillan K & O'Herlihy C (2001) Influence of persistent occiput posterior position on delivery outcome. *Obstetrics and Gynecology* **98**(6): 1027–1031.

Impy L & O'Herlihy C (1998) First delivery after caesarean delivery for strictly defined cephalopelvic disproportion. *Obstetrics and Gynecology* 92(5): 799–803.

Impy L, Hobson J & O'Herlihy C (2000) Graphic analysis of actively managed labour: prospective computation of progress in 500 consecutive nulliparous women in spontaneous labour at term. *American Journal of Obstetrics and Gynecology* 183(2): 438–443.

O'Driscoll K (1966) Rupture of the uterus. *Proceedings of the Royal Society of Medicine* 59: 65.

O'Driscoll K & Foley M (1983) Correlation of decrease in perinatal mortality and increase in caesarean section rates. *Obstetrics and Gynecology* 61: 1–5.

O'Driscoll K, Foley M, MacDonald D & Stronge J (1988) Cesarean section and perinatal outcome: response from the House of Horne. *American Journal of Obstetrics and Gynecology* 158: 449–452.

Stronge J, McQuillan K, Robson MS & Johnson H (1996) Factors affecting mode of delivery in labour following a single previous birth by caesarean section. *Journal of Obstetrics and Gynaecology* 16: 353–357.

Turner MJ, Rasmussen MJ, Boylan PC, MacDonald D & Stronge JM (1990) The influence of birth weight on labor in nulliparas. *Obstetrics and Gynecology* 76: 159–162.

Index